Firelands Regional Medical Center
School of Nursing Library
1912 Hayes Ave, Sandusky, OH 44870

W9-BIE-177

DOORWAY THOUGHTS

Cross-Cultural Health Care for Older Adults

Volume 2

Ethnogeriatrics Committee,
American Geriatrics Society

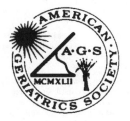

JONES AND BARTLETT PUBLISHERS
Sudbury, Massachusetts
BOSTON   TORONTO   LONDON   SINGAPORE

Jones and Bartlett Publishers

World Headquarters
Jones and Bartlett Publishers
40 Tall Pine Drive
Sudbury, MA 01776
978-443-5000
info@jbpub.com
www.jbpub.com

Jones and Bartlett Publishers Canada
6339 Ormindale Way
Mississauga, Ontario L5V 1J2
Canada

Jones and Bartlett Publishers International
Barb House, Barb Mews
London W6 7PA
United Kingdom

American Geriatrics Society

Executive Vice President: Linda Hiddeman Barondess
Manager, Governance and Public Policy: Julie Zaharatos, MPH
Senior Consultant: Jill Epstein, MA

The Empire State Building
350 Fifth Avenue, Suite 801
New York, NY 10118
(212) 308-1414
www.americangeriatrics.org

Jones and Bartlett's books and products are available through most bookstores and online booksellers. To contact Jones and Bartlett Publishers directly, call 800-832-0034, fax 978-443-8000, or visit our website, www.jbpub.com.

Substantial discounts on bulk quantities of Jones and Bartlett's publications are available to corporations, professional associations, and other qualified organizations. For details and specific discount information, contact the special sales department at Jones and Bartlett via the above contact information or send an email to specialsales@jbpub.com.

PRODUCTION CREDITS

Chief Executive Officer: Clayton Jones
Chief Operating Officer: Don W. Jones, Jr.
President, Higher Education and Professional Publishing: Robert W. Holland, Jr.
V.P., Sales and Marketing: William J. Kane
V.P., Design and Production: Anne Spencer
V.P., Manufacturing and Inventory Control: Therese Connell

Publisher, Public Safety Group: Kimberly Brophy
Associate Editor: Janet Morris
Production Editor: Karen C. Ferreira
Photo Researcher: Christine McKeen
Cover and Text Design: Anne Spencer
Composition: NK Graphics
Printing and Binding: Malloy

All rights reserved. No part of the material protected by this copyright may be reproduced or utilized in any form, electronic or mechanical, including photocopying, recording, or by any information storage and retrieval system, without written permission from the copyright owner.

The procedures and protocols in this book are based on the most current recommendations of responsible medical sources. The American Geriatrics Society and the publisher, however, make no guarantee as to, and assume no responsibility for the correctness, sufficiency, or completeness of such information or recommendations. Other or additional safety measures may be required under particular circumstances.

This textbook is intended as a guide to the appropriate procedures to be employed when rendering medical care to the geriatric population. It is not intended as a statement of the standards of care required in any particular situation, because the circumstances and the patient's physical condition can vary widely from one case to another. Nor is it intended that this textbook shall in any way advise medical personnel concerning legal authority to perform activities or procedures discussed. Such local determination should be made only with the aid of legal counsel.

Notice: The patients described in the Case Studies throughout this text are fictitious.

© 2006 by American Geriatrics Society

ISBN-10: 0-7637-4355-0   ISBN-13: 978-0-7637-4355-0

Library of Congress Cataloging-in-Publication Data
Doorway thoughts: cross-cultural health care for older adults / from the Ethnogeriatrics Steering Committee of the American Geriatrics Society.
    p. ; cm.
  Includes bibliographic references and index.
  ISBN 0-7637-3338-5 (pbk. : alk. paper)
  1. Minority aged--Medical care--Cross-cultural studies. 2. Minority aged--Health and hygiene. 3. Aged--Cross-cultural studies. 4. Gerontology--Cross-cultural studies. 5. Minority aged--Services for.
  [DNLM: 1. Geriatrics--United States. 2. Cross-Cultural Comparison--United States. 3. Health Services for the Aged--United States. 4. Minority Groups--Aged--United States. 5. Professional-Patient Relations--Aged--United States. WT 30 D691 2004] I. Title: Cross-cultural health care for older adults. II. American Geriatrics Society. Ethnogeriatrics Steering Committee.
  RA564.8.D66 2004
  362.6'1'0973--dc22
6048   2004004946

Printed in the United States of America
10 09 08 07 06   10 9 8 7 6 5 4 3 2 1

Doorway Thoughts Editorial Board

Series Editorial Committee

Reva N. Adler, MD, MPH, FRCPC, **Editor**
Clinical Associate Professor,
Associate, Center for International Health
Department of Medicine
University of British Columbia
Medical Director, STAT Centre
Vancouver Coastal Health Authority
Vancouver General Hospital and Health
Sciences Centre
Vancouver, British Columbia, Canada

Cynthia X. Pan, MD
Associate Professor, Brookdale Department of
Geriatrics and Adult Development
Director of Education, Hertzberg Palliative Care
Institute
Mount Sinai School of Medicine
New York, New York, USA

Sharon A. Brangman, MD, FACP, AGSF
Professor, Division Chief, Geriatric Medicine
SUNY Upstate Medical University
Syracuse, New York, USA

Gwen Yeo, PhD
Director, Stanford Geriatric Education Center
California Council on Gerontology and
Geriatrics
Stanford University School of Medicine
Palo Alto, California, USA

Contributors

Chapter 1: Introduction
Reva N. Adler, MD, MPH, FRCPC
Clinical Associate Professor,
Associate, Center for International Health
Department of Medicine
University of British Columbia
Medical Director, STAT Centre
Vancouver Coastal Health Authority
Vancouver General Hospital and Health
Sciences Centre
Vancouver, British Columbia, Canada

Chapter 2: Older Arab Americans
Sonia L. Salari, PhD
Assistant Professor
Family and Consumer Studies
University of Utah
Salt Lake City, Utah, USA

Chapter 2: Older Arab Americans
Hashim Balubaid, MB, ChBSSC-Med
Consultant, Geriatric Medicine
King Abdulaziz Medical City Riyadh,
Saudi Arabia
Fellowships in Geriatric Medicine and in
Palliative Care Medicine, Vancouver, British
Columbia, Canada

Chapter 3: Older Cambodian Americans
Barbara W.K. Yee, PhD
Professor and Chair
University of Hawaii at Manoa
Dept. of Family and Consumer Sciences
Honolulu, Hawaii, USA

Chapter 3: Older Cambodian Americans
Yani Rose Keo
Cambodian Elder
Refuge Services Alliance
Houston, Texas, USA

Chapter 4: Older Filipino Americans
Melen R. McBride, PhD, RN
Associate Director
Stanford Geriatric Education Center
School of Medicine, Stanford University
Palo Alto, California, USA

Chapter 4: Older Filipino Americans
Rena Nora, MD
Clinical Professor
Department of Psychiatry
University of Nevada School of Medicine
Las Vegas, Nevada, USA

Chapter 4: Older Filipino Americans
Vyjeyanthi S. Periyakoil, MD
Director, VA Geriatrics Clinic
Associate Medical Director, Palo Alto VA
Hospice Care Center
Palo Alto, California, USA

Chapter 5: Older Haitian Americans
Monica Stallworth, MD, MPH, CMD
Medical Director, Neville Center at Fresh Pond
Nursing and Rehabilitation Center
Faculty, Harvard Division on Aging
Geriatrician, Harvard Medical School
Cambridge Health Alliance
Boston, Massachusetts, USA

Chapter 6: Older Korean Americans
Linda Sohn, MD, MPH
Assistant Clinical Professor Medicine/Geriatrics
UCLA School of Medicine
Associate Director, Sepulveda VA NHCU
Sepulveda, California, USA

Chapter 7: Older Pakistani Americans
Amna B. Buttar, MD, MS
Clinical Associate Professor of Medicine
University of Wisconsin Medical School
Madison, Wisconsin, USA

Chapter 7: Older Pakistani Americans
Jennifer C. Mendez, PhD
Institute of Gerontology
Wayne State University
Detroit, Michigan, USA

Chapter 7: Older Pakistani Americans
Vyjeyanthi S. Periyakoil, MD
Director, VA Geriatrics Clinic
Associate Medical Director, Palo Alto VA
Hospice Care Center
Palo Alto, California, USA

Chapter 8: Older Portuguese Americans
Ana Perry Nava, PhD
Psychotherapist, Portuguese Mental Health
Clinic, Cambridge Health Alliance
Director of Clinical Services, Massachusetts
Alliance of Portuguese Speakers (MAPS)
Cambridge, Massachusetts, USA

Chapter 8: Older Portuguese Americans
Helena Santos-Martins, MD
Medical Director, East Cambridge Health
Center, Cambridge Health Alliance
Instructor of Medicine
Harvard Medical School
Cambridge, Massachusetts, USA

*Chapter 9: Older Russian-Speaking
Americans*
Karen Aroian, PhD, RN
Katharine E. Faville Professor of Nursing
Research
Wayne State University
Detroit, Michigan, USA

*Chapter 9: Older Russian-Speaking
Americans*
Galina Khatutsky, MS
Research Associate
Aging, Disability, and Long Term Care Program
RTI International
Belmont, Massachusetts, USA

*Chapter 9: Older Russian-Speaking
Americans*
Alexandra Dashevskaya, MA, MS
Manager, Bilingual Services Program
Hebrew Rehabilitation Center
Roslindale, Massachusetts, USA

Medical Editor

Barbara B. Reitt, PhD, ELS(D), Reitt Editing
Services

Doorway Thoughts: Cross-Cultural Health Care for Older Adults, Volume 1:

Introduction to Cross-Cultural Health Care for Older Adults

Older American Indians and Alaska Natives

Older Hispanic Americans

Older African Americans

Older Vietnamese Americans

Older Asian Indian Americans

Older Japanese Americans

Older Chinese Americans

ISBN: 0-7637-3338-5 © 2004

CONTENTS

Acknowledgments

The editor and editorial committee wish to thank everyone involved in the development of this second volume of *Doorway Thoughts:* the authors, who gave so generously of their time and experience in writing each chapter; the Ethnogeriatrics Committee of the American Geriatrics Society (AGS), whose hard work and dedication paved our way; the AGS Board of Directors, committee chairs, and members for their invaluable comments and suggestions; Jerry C. Johnson, MD, AGSF, for his expert assistance from the onset of this series and David Reuben, MD, AGSF, for his continued enthusiasm and promotion of the project; our medical editor, Barbara B. Reitt, PhD, ELS(D); and Jill Epstein, Julie Zaharatos, and the AGS staff, who have been essential to the success of this volume.

Editor: Reva N. Adler, MD, MPH, FRCPC
Editorial Committee: Sharon Brangman, MD, FACP, AGSF; Cynthia Pan, MD; and Gwen Yeo, PhD

Preface

Cultural diversity in North America is increasing annually. In 2000, the percentage of Americans reporting European ancestry decreased considerably, while the percentage of Americans born in Latin America and Asia rose significantly. In developing *Doorway Thoughts*, Volume 2 (DT2), the Editorial Board expanded on the first volume by writing about two general groups of older Americans: those whose populations are rapidly increasing, such as Filipino, Vietnamese, Korean, Pakistani, Haitian, and Arab Americans, and those with distinct cultural traditions in a stable, significant population base in the United States, such as Portuguese and Russian-speaking Americans. The Editorial Board hopes that readers will find these chapters helpful in everyday practice.

In *DT2*, we have added a new topic heading, Home Care and Food. As the emphasis on home-based health services in North America increases and as palliative care enters the mainstream of older adult care, several readers of the first volume requested this addition in order to optimize the services they are providing in intercultural settings. We hope that readers will find this addition both informative and useful, and we welcome feedback for improvements to future volumes.

Organizations such as the American College of Physicians, the Accreditation Council for Graduate Medical Education, the American Academy of Family Physicians, the American Nurses Association, the American Physical Therapy Association, the American Occupational Therapy Association, and the National Association of Social Workers have all highlighted cultural literacy and improvements in minority health services as priority practice areas. *DT2* has been designed to be of use in a variety of settings, including clinical practice, clinical education, continuing professional education, staff in-service education, and quality-improvement activities. It is our hope that these volumes will serve as a succinct and useful tool for a variety of our colleagues in the health professions—in their everyday practice, as well as in workplace, university, and postgraduate educational activities.

The American Geriatrics Society and the Editorial Board of *Doorway Thoughts* look forward to publishing *Doorway*

Thoughts, Volume 3, in the spring of 2008. This third volume will focus on a collection of topics relevant to intercultural care, including health literacy, approaches to clinician education, and the interface between spirituality and health decision making.

Finally, we hope that readers will take the time to explore recommended resources in cross-cultural care that are available on the World Wide Web. Examples include the Web site of the American Medical Student Association entitled Cultural Competency in Medicine (www.amsa.org/programs/gpit/cultural.cfm), the EthnoMed Web site of the University of Washington Harborview Medical Center (ethnomed.org), the Web site of the Collaborative on Ethnogeriatric Education entitled Curriculum in Ethnogeriatrics (www.stanford.edu/group/ethnoger), the site of the Stanford Geriatric Education Center entitled Improving Communication with Elders of Different Cultures (sgec.stanford.edu/training/cultures.html), and the site of OnLok Senior Health and Stanford Geriatric Education Center entitled Diversity, Healing and Health Care (www.gasi.org/diversity.htm), a resource for clinicians who work with patients whose religions and cultures are different from their own.

Reva N. Adler, MD, MPH, FRCPC

Sharon A. Brangman, MD, FACP, AGSF

Gwen Yeo, PhD

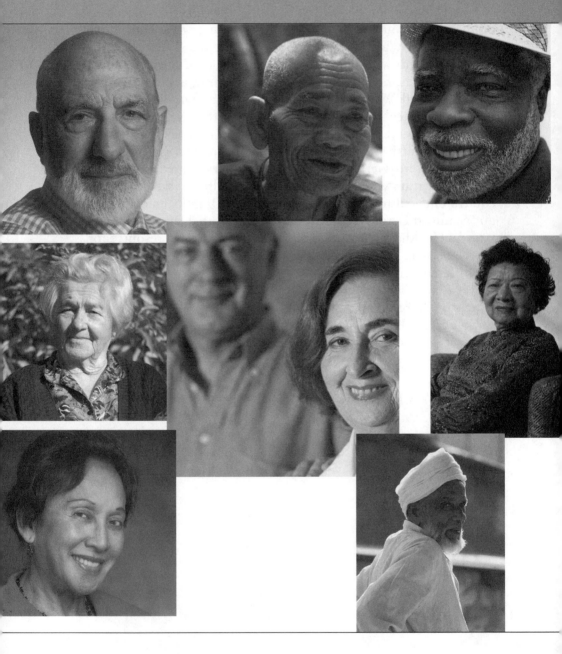

CHAPTER I

Cross-Cultural Health Care for Older Adults

Doorway Thoughts

The key concepts discussed in this series are *doorway thoughts*—factors that the culturally competent practitioner reflects upon before walking through the doorway of any examining, consultation, or hospital room. These factors can shape intercultural health care encounters and relationships for good or for ill. Cultural and historical facts and issues relating to the members of an entire minority group can be in play in any cross-cultural encounter or relationship. The practitioner should be sensitive to the possibility that they may affect relations with individual patients and families and may also affect patients' willingness or ability to understand, accept, and adhere to prescribed regimens.

The quality of any encounter between a clinician and a patient from different ethnic or cultural backgrounds depends on the clinician's skill and sensitivity. Questions about the individual patient's attitudes and beliefs should be worked naturally and carefully into the clinical interview. Remember that no culture is monolithic. Attitudes and beliefs vary widely from one individual to another within a single cultural group. Prior familiarity with a patient's cultural background will not suffice, because it is inaccurate to assume that a person's outlook is inflexibly linked to his or her cultural heritage. The concepts presented in this text are intended to serve as guides in choosing appropriate questions, rather than as a rigid list of cultural attributes or clinical scenarios.

Cultural and historical facts and issues relating to the members of an entire minority group can be in play in any cross-cultural encounter or relationship.

Preferred Terms for Cultural Identity

The terms referring to specific cultural or ethnic groups can change over time, and individuals in any one group do not always agree on the terminology that is appropriate. It is important to learn what the individual patient's preferred term is for his or her cultural identity and to use that terminology in conversation with the patient, as well as in his or her health records.

Attitudes regarding the appropriate degree of formality in a health care encounter differ widely among cultural groups.

Formality

Attitudes regarding the appropriate degree of formality in a health care encounter differ widely among cultural groups. Learning what a new patient's preferences are with regard to formality and allowing that preference to shape the relationship is always advisable. Initially, a more formal approach is likely to be appropriate.

Addressing the Patient

The patient's correct title (e.g., Dr., Reverend, Mr., Mrs., Ms., Miss) and his or her surname should be used unless and until he or she requests a more casual form of address. Another important issue is to determine the correct pronunciation of the person's name.

Addressing the Health Provider

It is also important to learn how the patient would prefer to address the clinician and to allow his or her preference to prevail. For example, in some cultures, trust in the physician depends on the physician assuming an authoritative role, and informality would undermine the patient's trust. This is an aspect of the clinical relationship where the clinician's personal preferences can be relinquished.

Language and Literacy

- What language does this individual feel most comfortable speaking? Will a medical interpreter be needed?
- Does this patient read and write English? Have a different primary language? If so, which one(s)?

- If the patient is not literate, does he or she have access to someone who can assist at home with written instructions?

It is worthwhile to consider these questions early in the health care relationship to determine whether interpretation services are needed and to make certain that communication with the patient is effective. The clinician should remember that even those who use English fluently may wish to discuss complicated issues in their native language. If possible, the use of family members, especially children, as interpreters should be avoided to decrease the chance of lack of critical vocabulary in one or both languages and to avert censoring of information. It is the clinician's responsibility to explain medical terms and to ask the patient for explanations of any cultural or foreign terms that are unfamiliar.

Respectful Nonverbal Communication

Body position and motion are interpreted differently from one cultural group to another. Specific hand gestures, facial expression, physical contact, and eye contact can hold different meanings for the patient and the clinician when their cultural backgrounds differ. The clinician should watch for particular body language cues that appear to be significant and that might be linked to cultural norms that are important to the patient, in order to cultivate a sensitivity to the conditions that make the flow of communication easy and effective.

Early in a relationship with a patient or when in doubt, the clinician should adopt conservative body language (assume a calm demeanor; avoid expressive extremes such as very vigorous handshakes, a loud and hearty voice, many hand gestures, or, on the other hand, an impassive facial expression or standing at a distance). Remain alert for signals that the person is comfortable or uncomfortable. Shaking hands, especially with members of the opposite sex, or sustained eye contact is not seen as respectful or appropriate in various cultures. Directly asking the patient questions about body language may also help. It is very important to avoid making negative judgments about a patient that are rooted in unconscious cultural assumptions about the meaning of his or her gestures, facial expressions, or body language.

Body position and motion are interpreted differently from one cultural group to another.

The distance from others that individuals find comfortable varies, depending in part on their cultural background. The clinician should determine what distance seems to be the most comfortable for each patient and, whenever practicable, allow the patient's preference to establish the optimal distance during the encounter.

Elephants in the Room

Are there any issues that are critical to the success of the health care encounter that are present but that go unspoken? The clinician must be alert for the possibility that such issues are indeed present. Examples include:

- a lack of trust in health care providers and the health care system
- a fear of medical research and experimentation
- fear of medications or their side effects
- unfamiliarity or discomfort with the Western biomedical belief system

In other chapters, these topics are covered in detail as they relate to specific cultural groups. In general, sensitivity to the possibility that such issues are in play is advised in all intercultural patient encounters.

History of Traumatic Experiences

Is the patient a refugee or survivor of violence or genocide? Are family members missing or dead? Have patients or family members been tortured? Such experiences could negatively affect the health care encounter without the clinician's knowledge unless relevant questions are included among standard questions about the patient's history.

It is important for clinicians to remember that in some historical periods and jurisdictions, health care providers participated in torture and genocide.

It is important for clinicians to remember that in some historical periods and jurisdictions, health care providers participated in torture and genocide. For example, during World War II, Nazi medical personnel were responsible in concentration camps for selecting individuals for gassing, supervising the gassing process, and administering lethal injections to inmates in "hospitals." The methods and tools of torture employed have sometimes resembled legitimate clinical procedures and tools. Patients surviving such experiences may not feel safe in medical or governmental settings, and contact with all clinicians may invoke feelings of vulnerability, fear, panic, or anger. Great sensitivity is necessary in providing health care for these individuals.

Immigration Status

Some individuals may be residing in North America without the protection of appropriate immigration documents. Clinicians may wish to assure each patient that information given within the medical encounter will be kept in the strictest confidence.

History of Immigration or Migration

The history of the movements of a whole ethnic or cultural group can affect the attitudes and behavior of individuals in that group for generations, even when they themselves have not immigrated to North America. Understanding the specific migration history of a person often provides insight into the key life transitions informing his or her outlook. In addition, knowing how a person came to reside in North America can be important. The time and effort the clinician invests in learning more about a minority group's history and current situation can be repaid not only in a better relationship with the individual patient but also in an enhanced appreciation of the factors affecting clinical relationships with all patients from that group.

Acculturation

Acculturation is defined as a process in which members of one cultural group adopt the beliefs and behaviors of another group. Acculturation of a group may be evidenced by changes in language preference, adoption of common attitudes and values, and gradual loss of separate ethnic identification. Although acculturation typically occurs when a minority group adopts the habits and language patterns of a dominant group, acculturation may also be reciprocal between groups.

It is essential to keep principles of acculturation in mind during any intercultural health encounter. Begin by determining how long a person has lived in North America and whether he or she was born here. However, remember that the degree to which the person is acculturated to Western customs and attitudes is the consequence of many factors and not just of the number of years since he or she immigrated. Older adults who follow the traditions of their cultural group may have been born outside of the United States or Canada, may be recent arrivals to the continent, or may even be lifelong North American residents.

A patient's level of acculturation may greatly impact not only his or her health behavior but also preferences in end-of-life planning and decision making. Acculturation can also be an issue dividing family members; in addition, a person's resistance to or ease of acculturation may be a matter of pride or shame and guilt. Developing sensitivity about the issues of acculturation for one's older minority patients is a key element in effective intercultural health care. Asking patients directly about their adherence to cultural traditions can be useful.

Tradition and Health Beliefs

People from non-Western cultural groups may not conceive of illness in Western terms. Some may have highly developed concepts of the causes of health and disease that are incompatible with the concepts that form the foundations of Western medicine. Non-Western paradigms include beliefs that illnesses have spiritual causation or are the result of imbalance among essential physical components or bodily humors, or that they are caused by a person's actions in past lives, to name but a few.

People from non-Western cultural groups may not conceive of illness in Western terms.

Patients may be making unexamined assumptions that are based on traditional beliefs, and these can cause confusion or create misunderstanding. The more the clinician knows about specific traditions, the more he or she can avoid such problems.

In addition, the clinician should remain alert to the possibility that patients holding such beliefs may be using alternative remedies (e.g., rituals, herbal preparations) that they may not mention. Questions about such practices should be included among other questions about the patient's history. It is unrealistic to expect that a patient will simply "adapt" to Western approaches to health and health care, just as it is impractical to expect the clinician to accept a new paradigm of wellness and disease. Clinical communication and efficacy will be enhanced when the patient and provider make an effort to negotiate a common understanding of causation, diagnosis, and treatment for a specific health problem while maintaining respect for the beliefs and constructs of both individuals.

Use of North American Health Services

Some minority patients may feel comfortable in customary North American health care settings. Explanations for the discomfort, distrust, or uneasiness of some include lack of familiarity with Western practices, dissatisfying previous encounters with the health care system, or the belief that insensitivity or discrimination is inevitable for anyone in the cultural or ethnic group. Such feelings may result from having been stereotyped or treated insensitively or even unfairly by health professionals in the past. Sensitive exploration of these issues with patients is often both worthwhile and necessary. Individual chapters in this text provide suggestions for possible approaches to patients in specific cultural groups. Generally, the clinician meeting a new patient from an ethnic or cultural minority group should be alert for signs of guardedness that signal an underlying lack of comfort or trust.

Home Care and Food

Food and nutrition are central issues in every culture, and they may take on even more importance when one is sick. This is true not only because of individual and community preferences but also because each culture believes that certain foods or preparations may have a beneficial or harmful effect in the face of illness. While in a hospital or residential facility, people can find it difficult to control what they eat. Such details can have a magnified impact on an older adult's sense of well-being, as well as on his or her willingness to adhere to a clinician's recommendations. When working in multicultural settings, clinicians are advised to ask gentle but direct questions regarding preferences and beliefs about food and intake and to incorporate such preferences in the treatment plan when possible. At times, this will also mean working with family members, who may be expected by patients to provide food and meals not only in the home but also in the hospital or residential facility.

Similarly, every culture has rituals regarding proper etiquette while at home. These may be as simple as removing shoes at the doorway or they may be complex as when spiritual or religious rituals are involved. The culturally sensitive clinician providing home care will enter a new patient's home with an air of inquisitive respect and will gently ask for permission and agreement before initiating each aspect of the clinical encounter.

Home care issues are particularly important for elders from diverse cultures because there is a strong preference by many elders and their families from non-European backgrounds to care for dependent and ill older members at home rather than in institutional long-term-care settings.

Individual chapters in this volume describe key issues regarding food and home care for elders in the cultural group being discussed. As with all aspects of cross-cultural care, an approach of mutual curiosity and deference when getting to know patients will optimize satisfaction and efficacy during the clinical encounter, whatever the setting.

Culture-Specific Health Risks

Epidemiologic and medical research has identified numerous differences among ethnic and cultural populations with regard to specific health risks. The clinician who treats many patients from a specific group is advised to make every effort to stay abreast of the latest findings in relevant areas. In the individual chapters of this text, the prevailing thinking about such risks for each group is reviewed.

Approaches to Decision Making

The influence of specific cultures on approaches to health decision making has been the subject of many studies. Western bioethics emphasize individual autonomy in all health decisions, but for many other cultures, decision making is family- or community-centered. Autonomy principles allow competent persons to involve others in their health decisions or to cede those rights to a proxy decision maker. The clinician should ask patients if they prefer to make their own health decisions or if they would prefer to involve or defer to others in the decision-making process. Some may wish to assign the decision-making authority wholly to another individual or a group. In some cultures, the definition of family may include *fictive kin* (people who are considered family despite having no blood relation). In families where the degree of acculturation of the generations differs, the older person may defer to or depend on younger relatives even though the tradition might suggest that the reverse would occur.

> *Western bioethics emphasize individual autonomy in all health decisions, but for many other cultures, decision making is family- or community-centered.*

Establishing an understanding of each patient's decision-making preferences early in the clinical relationship will, in most instances, promote better communication and avert the difficulties inherent in trying to address the issues at a time of crisis. When the patient's and clinician's cultural backgrounds differ, careful exploration of the issues is all the more important because the clinician cannot proceed if clinician and patient are not starting from a point of shared understanding.

Disclosure and Consent

Cultural attitudes toward truth telling and disclosure of terminal diagnoses vary widely. In some cultures, it is commonly believed that patients should not be informed of a terminal diagnosis, because this may be injurious to health or hasten death. Obtaining informed consent in such cases may prove to be difficult. There is no consensus in bioethics concerning the rigorous application of full clinical disclosure in every situation. However, it is generally agreed that incorporating a patient's beliefs concerning disclosure and truth telling into clinical planning whenever possible is desirable. Some patients may prefer not to know if they are terminally ill and ask that family members or other caregivers receive all diagnostic information and make all treatment decisions. It is

> *Cultural attitudes toward truth telling and disclosure of terminal diagnoses vary widely.*

advisable to explore each patient's preferences regarding disclosure of serious clinical findings early in the clinical relationship and to reconfirm these wishes at intervals.

Gender Issues

Each culture has intricate traditions and structures with regard to gender roles. Societies seemingly based on the same patriarchal or matriarchal model may vary widely in their expressions of the model. A person's gender influences the sorts of experiences he or she has had, not only within the family but in the community and health care system as well. Another level of complexity may be added to health care encounters when an older adult's group struggles with conflicting traditional and contemporary views on gender roles. Cultural norms for men and women can profoundly influence their health behavior and their expectations of the health care interaction; these norms for the genders vary widely from one culture to another. Many societies with clear and strongly differentiated gender roles do not condone cross-sex patient-provider (or interpreter) interactions. These norms also affect decision making, disclosure, and consent.

Cultural norms for men and women can profoundly influence their health behavior and their expectations of the health care interaction.

It is highly advisable for the clinician to explore each patient's attitudes regarding the interplay among gender, autonomy, and personal decision making early in the patient-provider relationship, to confirm his or her preferences at intervals, and to follow the individual patient's wishes whenever possible.

End-of-Life Decision Making and Care Intensity

Culture is an important influence in a person's formation of his or her attitudes toward supportable quality of life, approach to suffering, and beliefs about medical feeding, life-prolonging treatments, and palliative care. Some cultures value a direct struggle for life in the face of death, and both patients and families will expect an intensive approach to treatment. Other cultures ardently avoid direct confrontation of death and dying and will prefer to leave such decisions to the clinician. Still others will take a direct approach to death and dying but will reject too aggressive an approach.

Research has shown that physicians and patients from shared cultural backgrounds have similar values in these areas; the implications of such findings for clinicians and patients from differing backgrounds are obviously important. Both physicians and patients bring their own attitudes and beliefs to any clinical encounter. It is important for clinicians to be aware of their personal views and cultural mind set when discussing end-of-life plans with patients and to respect patients' beliefs and preferences even when they are different from the clinician's beliefs.

In negotiating end-of-life directions with a patient whose background is different from his or her own, the clinician must listen especially carefully to the patient's goals and concerns and exert every effort to avoid making culture-based assumptions that do not apply. For example, the assumption that "no one would want to live in that condition" or that "everyone would want treatment in this situation" is likely to be faulty. To ensure that end-of-life plans and decisions reflect an individual's rights and wishes, the clinician must strive to understand the older person's overall approach to life and death, and, as far as possible, provide care that is congruent with that approach.

In the chapters on specific cultural or ethnic groups, the authors provide data from the health services literature regarding the general preferences of a group for end-of-life decisions, life-sustaining care, and advance directives. This information is intended to provide general guidance rather than absolute rules for clinicians when they are discussing end-of-life issues with patients and caregivers from different cultural backgrounds.

Use of Advance Directives

The use of advance directives and health care proxies has become more common in the past 20 years, but research indicates that the use of written directives may be more common among older persons in the dominant North American culture than among older persons in minority cultural groups. It is advisable in intercultural situations, when discussing attitudes and beliefs regarding written directives with a patient, to be sensitive to the possibility that some minority older persons will prefer to use alternatives—verbal directives or directives dictated to family members or others—and others will need to avoid any such discussion so as to observe proscriptions against talking about death. In view of the fact that preferences for care intensity may also differ according to cultural background, patients should also be given the opportunity to indicate the interventions they do want as well as those they do not want in any written or verbal directive used.

Cultural Competence: A Final Word

There is no gold standard definition of cultural competence. Most definitions emphasize a careful coordination of individual behavior, organizational policy, and system design to facilitate mutually respectful and effective cross-cultural interactions.

Cultural competence combines attitudes, knowledge base, acquired skills, and behavior—it is an approach, not a technique. Cultural competence is not a form of "political correctness." Ideally, it is a nuanced understanding of the determining role that culture plays in each person's life and of the impact culture has on every health care encounter, for both the clinician and the patient.

Cultural competence cannot be achieved exclusively by reading, but we hope that the *Doorway Thoughts* volumes will provide clinicians who care for older persons from all minority groups with basic information and a foundation for further investigation. We encourage clinicians to view each intercultural encounter as an opportunity to learn more, not only about the individual patient and his or her culture, but also about themselves. The authors also recommend that clinicians learn more about the impact of culture on health decisions by reading the publications listed in the bibliographies, exploring available Web sites, and attending workshops. We also urge clinicians to work with the entire interdisciplinary health care team, including administrators, to promote cultural competence in the health care organizations where they practice. Finally, we encourage clinician educators to develop their own teaching materials and educational programs specifically designed to meet the needs of specific communities.

> *Cultural competence combines attitudes, knowledge base, acquired skills, and behavior.*

Reva N. Adler, MD, MPH, FRCPC

References

Adelman RD, Greene MG, Charon R, Friedman E. Content of elderly patient-physician interviews in the medical primary care encounter. *Communication Research* 1992;19(3):370–380.

Adler RN, Kamel HK, eds. *Doorway Thoughts: Cross-Cultural Health Care for Older Adults*. Vol. 1. Sudbury, MA: Jones and Bartlett Publishers; 2004.

American Medical Student Association. Cultural competency in medicine. Available at: www.amsa.org/programs/gpit/cultural.cfm (accessed December 2005).

Anderson NB, Bulatas RA, Cohen B, eds. *Critical Perspectives on Racial and Ethnic Differences in Health in Late Life*. Washington, DC: National Academies Press for the National Research Council; 2004.

Beisecker AE. Aging and the desire for information and input in medical decisions: patient consumerism in medical encounters. *Gerontologist* 1988;28(3): 330–335.

Beisecker AE, Beisecker TD. Patient information-seeking behaviors when communicating with doctors. *Med Care* 1990;28(1):19–28.

Blackhall LJ, Murphy ST, Frank G, et al. Ethnicity and attitudes toward patient autonomy. *JAMA* 1995;274(10):820–825.

Braun KL, Pietsch JH, Blanchette PL, eds. *Cultural Issues in End-of-Life Decision Making*. Thousand Oaks, CA: Sage; 2000.

Burke G. Ethics and medical decision-making. *Prim Care* 1980;7(4):615–624.

Caralis P, Davis B, Wright K, et al. The influence of ethnicity and race on attitudes toward advance directives, life-prolonging treatments, and euthanasia. *J Clin Ethics* 1993;4(2):155–165.

Charles C, Gould M, Chambers L, et al. How was your hospital stay? Patients' reports about their care in Canadian hospitals. *CMAJ* 1994;150(11):1813–1822.

Clark JA, Potter DA, McKinlay JB. Bringing social structure back into clinical decision making. *Soc Sci Med* 1991;32(8):853–866.

Cotton P. Talk to people about dying—they can handle it, say geriatricians and patients. *JAMA* 1993;269(3):321–322.

Eleazer GP, Hornung C, Egbert C, et al. The relationship between ethnicity and advance directives in a frail older population. *J Am Geriatr Soc* 1996;44(8):938–943.

Emanuel EJ, Emanuel LL. Four models of the physician-patient relationship. *JAMA* 1992;267(16):2221–2226.

Finucane TE, Shumway JM, Powers RL, et al. Planning with elderly outpatients for contingencies of severe illness: a survey and clinical trial. *J Gen Intern Med* 1988;3(4):322–325.

Fox SA, Stein JA. The effect of physician-patient communication on mammography utilization by different ethnic groups. *Med Care* 1991;29(11):1065–1082.

Garrett JM, Harris RP, Norburn JK, et al. Life-sustaining treatments during terminal illness: who wants what? *J Gen Intern Med* 1993;8(7):361–368.

Goold SD, Arnold RM, Siminoff LA. Discussions about limiting treatment in a geriatric clinic. *J Am Geriatr Soc* 1993;41(3):277–281.

Green, JW. *Cultural Awareness in the Human Services: A Multi-Ethnic Approach.* Boston: Allyn and Bacon; 1998.

Hall JA, Roter DL, Katz NR. Meta-analysis of correlates of provider behavior in medical encounters. *Med Care* 1988;26(7):657–675.

Hare J, Nelson C. Will outpatients complete living wills? a comparison of two interventions. *J Gen Intern Med* 1991;6(1):41–46.

Harwood A, ed. *Ethnicity and Medical Care.* Cambridge, MA: Harvard University Press; 1981.

Haug MR. Doctor-patient relationships and the older patient. *J Gerontol* 1979;34(6):852–860.

Haug MR, Ory MG. Issues in elder patient-provider interactions. *Res Aging* 1987;9(1):39–44.

Helman CG. *Culture, Health and Illness: An Introduction for Health Professionals.* 3rd ed. Oxford, UK: Butterworth-Heinemann Ltd.; 1994.

High D. Advance directives and the elderly: a study of intervention strategies to increase use. *Gerontologist* 1993;33(3):342–349.

Hypertension Detection and Follow-up Program Cooperative Group. Five-year findings of the Hypertension Detection and Follow-up Program: II: mortality by race-sex and age. *JAMA* 1979;242(23):2572–2577.

Janofsky JS, Rovner BW. Prevalence of advance directives and guardianship in nursing home patients. *J Geriatr Psychiatry Neurol* 1993;6(4):214–216.

Jennings, B. Cultural diversity meets end-of-life decision making. *Hosp Health Netw* 1994;68(18):72.

Jensen J. Trust in doctor deters elderly from seeing other providers. *Mod Healthc* 1986;16(9):49–50.

Kalish RA, Reynolds DK. *Death and Ethnicity: A Psychocultural Study.* Los Angeles: University of Southern California Press; 1976.

Kim SS. Ethnic elders and American health care—a physician's perspective. *West J Med* 1983;139(6):885–891.

Klessig J. The effect of values and culture on life-support decisions. *West J Med* 1992;157(3):316–322.

Levy DR. White doctors and black patients: influence of race on the doctor-patient relationship. *Pediatr* 1985;75(4):639–643.

Lipson, JG, Dibble SL, Minarik PA, eds. *Culture and Nursing Care: A Pocket Guide.* San Francisco: UCSF Nursing Press; 1996.

Marcus AC, Reeder LG, Jordan LA, et al. Monitoring health status, access to health care, and compliance behavior in a large urban community: a report from the Los Angeles health survey. *Med Care* 1980;18(3):253–265.

Morioka-Douglas N, Sachs T, Yeo G. Issues in the care of Afghan American elders: insights from the literature and a focus group. *J Cross Cult Gerontol* 2004;19:27–40.

Murphy S, Palmer J, Azen S, et al. Ethnicity and advance care directives. *J Law Med Ethics* 1996;24(2):108–117.

Palafox N, Warren A, eds. *Cross-Cultural Caring: A Handbook for Health Care Professionals in Hawaii*. Honolulu, HI: Transcultural Health Care Forum; 1980.

Reilly BM, Magnussen CR, Ross J, et al. Can we talk? Inpatient discussions about advance directives in a community hospital: attending physicians' attitudes, their inpatients' wishes, and reported experience. *Arch Intern Med* 1994;154(20):2299–2308.

Roter DL, Hall JA, Katz NR. Patient-physician communication: descriptive summary of the literature. Patient Education and Counseling 1988;12:99–119.

Rubin SM, Strull WM, Fialkow MF, et al. Increasing the completion of the durable power of attorney for health care: a randomized, controlled trial. *JAMA* 1994;271(3):209–212.

Sachs GA, Stocking CB, Miles SH. Empowerment of the older patient? a randomized, controlled trial to increase discussion and use of advance directives. *J Am Geriatr Soc* 1992;40(3):269–273.

Satcher D. Does race interfere with the doctor-patient relationship? *JAMA* 1973;223(13):1498–1499.

Schmerling RH, Bedell SE, Lilienfeld A, et al. Discussing cardiopulmonary resuscitation: a study of elderly outpatients. *J Gen Intern Med* 1988;3(4):317–321.

Schonwetter RS, Teasdale TA, Taffet G, et al. Educating the elderly: cardiopulmonary resuscitation decisions before and after intervention. *J Am Geriatr Soc* 1991;39(4):372–377.

Silverman H, Tuma P, Schaeffer M, et al. Implementation of the patient self-determination act in a hospital setting: an initial evaluation. *Arch Intern Med* 1995;155(3):502–510.

Smedley BD, Stith AY, Nelson AR, eds. *Unequal Treatment: Confronting Racial and Ethnic Disparities in Health Care*. Washington, DC: National Academies Press for the Institute of Medicine; 2003.

Smucker WD, Ditto PH, Moore KA, et al. Elderly outpatients respond favorably to a physician-initiated advance directive discussion. *J Am Board Fam Pract* 1993;6(5):473–482.

Szasz TS, Hollender MH. The basic models of the doctor-patient relationship. *Arch Intern Med* 1956;97:585–592.

Teno J, Fleishman J, Brock DW, et al. The use of formal prior directives among patients with HIV-related diseases. *J Gen Intern Med* 1990;5(6):490–494.

Terry M, Zweig S. Prevalence of advance directives and do-not-resuscitate orders in community nursing facilities. *Arch Fam Med* 1994;3(2):141–145.

Uhlmann RF, Pearlman RA, Cain KC. Understanding of elderly patients' resuscitation preferences by physicians and nurses. *West J Med* 1989;150(6):705–707.

University of Washington, Harborview Medical Center. EthnoMed. Available at: http:ethnomed.org (accessed December 2005).

Vaughn G, Kiyasu E, McCormick WC. Advance directive preferences among subpopulations of Asian nursing home residents in the Pacific Northwest. *J Am Geriatr Soc* 2000;48(5):554–557.

Veatch RM. Models for ethical medicine in a revolutionary age: what physician-patient roles foster the most ethical relationship? *Hastings Cent Rep* 1975;2(3):3–5.

Vukmir RB, Kremen R, Dehart DA, et al. Compliance with emergency department patient referral. *Am J Emerg Med* 1992;10(5):413–417.

Waitzkin H. Doctor-patient communication: clinical implications of social scientific research. *JAMA* 1984;252(17):2441–2446.

Ware JE Jr, Bayliss MS, Rogers WH, et al. Differences in 4-year health outcomes for elderly and poor, chronically ill patients treated in HMO and fee-for-service systems: results from the Medical Outcomes Study. *JAMA* 1996;276(13):1039–1047.

Yeo G, ed. Curriculum in ethnogeriatrics: core curriculum and ethnic specific modules. Available at: www.stanford.edu/group/ethnoger (accessed December 2005).

Yeo G, Hikoyeda N, McBride M, et al. *Cohort Analysis as a Tool in Ethnogeriatrics: Historical Profiles of Elders from Eight Ethnic Populations in the United States.* Stanford GEC Working Paper #12. Stanford, CA: Stanford Geriatric Education Center; 1998.

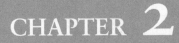

CHAPTER 2

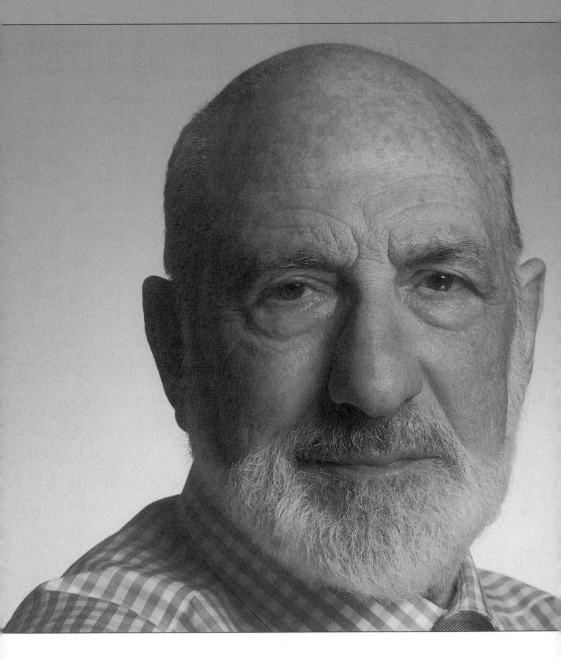

Older Arab Americans

Doorway Thoughts

Older Arab Americans are a diverse group with regard to citizenship, educational attainment, income, English-language skills, acculturation, immigration status, and religious views. As a group, Arab Americans are more likely to hold a graduate degree and earn an income above the national average. However, there are pockets of poverty in the population; lower economic status is usually associated with recent immigration and English-language difficulty. Recent U.S. and world events have focused attention on this ethnic group, sometimes resulting in stereotypes that negatively influence the quality of life for older Arab Americans and their families.

Preferred Cultural Terms

Older Arab Americans immigrated from or descend from one of 22 Arab-speaking countries. Although often confused as Arab Americans, those from Afghanistan, Iran, and Turkey are not included in this language-based ethnic classification. Despite various grades of skin coloration, persons of Arab origin are considered white. Not all older persons of Arab origin in the United States are Muslims; in fact, many are Christians, especially those who immigrated from or descend from Lebanon. The preferred forms of cultural reference for elders are *Arab American* or more specific linkages to a particular homeland, such as *Syrian American* or *Iraqi American.*

Formality of Address

Practitioners should be conservative about addressing older Arab Americans and use the patient's correct title and formal name. Physicians are usually highly regarded by Arab American elders and their families. Some, however, may have difficulty following

Practitioners should be conservative about addressing older Arab Americans and use the patient's correct title and formal name.

orders from nurses or allied health professionals, who may be considered to have lower authority. Physicians are encouraged to explain to Arab American elders the role of other health care professionals in the administration of medical procedures and their importance to achieving clinical goals.

Language and Literacy

Most older persons of Arab origin in the United States are first-generation immigrants; however, their English-language skills vary and are not necessarily linked to their immigration history. Proficient English speakers are likely to have been in the United States since they were younger adults; they may have obtained high levels of education and may be enjoying a relatively advantaged quality of life in North America. Whatever their immigration history, those who are bilingual have more opportunities in North America than do those who speak only Arabic. Older Arab immigrants who have arrived recently usually fall into the category of "followers of children." These newer arrivals may experience lower life satisfaction, largely because of their language difficulties. In some cases, newer older immigrants may not have been literate in their countries of origin, a fact that may further complicate their experience of North American life.

Respectful Nonverbal Communication

Many Arab Americans are comfortable with greeting the clinician with a handshake, but women who are Muslims may prefer not to shake hands with a male clinician. In addition, married Muslim women may prefer not to smile or maintain continuous eye contact with health care workers of either sex. An intense gaze from the clinician in this situation may cause discomfort for the patient. The astute clinician will be aware of the possibility that older Arab Americans will prefer more restrained body language and thus adopt a conservative approach when first encountering a new Arab patient.

Women who are Muslims may prefer not to shake hands with a male clinician.

Patterns of Immigration

Persons of Arab origins immigrated or descended from one of the Arabic-speaking countries, including Algeria, Bahrain, Egypt, Iraq, Jordan, Kuwait, Lebanon, Libya, Mauritania, Morocco, Oman, Palestine, Qatar, Saudi Arabia, Sudan, Syria, Tunisia, United Arab Emirates, and Yemen. The majority in the United States are Lebanese, Syrian, Palestinian, Egyptian, or Iraqi. There have been two major waves of immigration, the first from 1870 to World War II and the second from about 1946 to the present. Early immigrants were predominantly Christian; the majority of more-recent arrivals self-identify as Muslim. Settlements have concentrated in Los Angeles, Detroit, and New York City. Dearborn, Michigan, has the largest Arab American community in relation to the total population; 20 percent of the city's residents report Arab origins.

Persons who immigrated in later life are qualitatively different from those who have aged in this country. Specifically, migrants in later life not only may have language difficulties but are also more likely to be dependent on their adult children. They are also likely to be in a transitional phase of adaptation to life in North America and to have lower life satisfaction.

Tradition and Health Beliefs

Recent Arab immigrants may be hesitant or unwilling to schedule specific appointments and may see office visit timing as being flexible; they may arrive late or skip appointments, which can result in scheduling difficulties. These challenges may be compounded by unmet transportation needs, which are commonly reported in this population. In the Arab world, social interaction tends to be slower and less focused on punctuality than in the Western world, so clinicians treating Arab American elders may need to make adjustments that accommodate the Arab patient's conception of time.

> *Recent Arab immigrants may be hesitant or unwilling to schedule specific appointments and may see office visit timing as being flexible.*

Dietary issues are important for Muslim elders, because traditionally they do not drink alcohol, eat pork, or eat blood products. Halal methods should be used in preparing meats, but kosher preparation may be substituted. Halal meats require a particular type of slaughter, with blood draining out of the animal, prayer before the slaughter, supervision by religious personnel, and assurance that there has not been contamination with tools or surfaces used for nonhalal meats. Lard is another avoided ingredient; baked goods and crackers are therefore examined for their content before consumption. Hospitalized Muslims may prefer to eat food prepared by their families in order to maintain dietary standards.

Despite the concern over consumption of blood products, there is no prohibition against human blood transfusions. Giving and accepting blood are both acceptable for Muslims. However, there may be concern about forbidden substances in medicines or therapies, such as pork products, animal fats or gelatin, or alcohol.

Muslims may also resist eating or taking medications during the daytime hours of Ramadan, a holy month whose timing varies from year to year. Ramadan is considered a time for sacrifice, when worshipers practice self-control in order to become closer to God. Sick and elderly believers may be exempt from fasting during Ramadan, as some exceptions are made for frail individuals.

Elderly persons of Arab origin may subscribe to folk remedies and beliefs, although such practices are considered to be declining in significance. Beliefs may include concern about the evil eye; that is, those who are envious (usually of beautiful children) may have the power to inflict injury on the family. Folk prevention measures, which include religious measures, are taken to divert the evil spirit to prevent harm. The clinician working with Arab American elders is advised to explore these issues gently with their patients and to incorporate an understanding of traditional remedies into an overall care plan.

> *However, there may be concern about forbidden substances in medicines or therapies, such as pork products, animal fats or gelatin, or alcohol.*

Mental illness may be one of the most feared medical conditions among Arab Muslims. By tradition, psychiatric issues are thought to arise from a loss of faith in God or possession by evil. Those suffering from "madness" are likely to seek the help of a religious intermediary or a folk healer and may neglect formal medical care. Among elderly persons of Arab origin and their families, mental illness may be considered a secret to be minimized, covered up, or denied.

Arab Americans may view preventive medical treatment as less important than treatment of acute symptoms of illness and injury. They may expect prescription drugs to address their symptoms, but once symptoms subside, they

> *Mental illness may be one of the most feared medical conditions among Arab Muslims.*

may discontinue their prescribed regimen. Clinicians should be aware of this possibility when prescribing medications to Arab American elders and provide an explanation of why extended medication use is necessary. Clinician-patient negotiation may be necessary to promote adherence to long-term drug regimens.

In the Arab tradition, family members are obligated to visit and bring gifts to hospitalized elderly persons. Depending on the patient's and family's level of acculturation, Arab family members may not wish to adhere to family visitation restrictions in the hospital setting.

Culture-Specific Health Risks

Arab American elders in general enjoy good health; relatively few report functional impairments. Health conditions disproportionately found in those of Arab origin include hypertension, hypercholesterolemia, and Type 2 diabetes mellitus. These health problems are noted to worsen as immigrants have increasing tenure in the United States. This phenomenon has been linked to American trends in dietary intake, which includes more sugars, meats, and processed grains, and fewer raw fruits and vegetables than diets in the Arab countries. In the Arab American community, there is diversity with regard to adoption of Western dietary practices; Yemeni immigrants are reported to retain a more traditional Arab diet than some other Arab immigrant groups. In addition, many people in the Middle East walk a great deal more than Americans do, and regular exercise may become less common for immigrants who have settled in the United States.

> *Health conditions disproportionately found in those of Arab origin include hypertension, hypercholesterolemia, and Type 2 diabetes mellitus.*

Elephants in the Room

Arab Americans tend to trust science and the medical profession, and they may even show an exaggerated respect for the powers and authority of a physician. Even so, as noted, Arab American elders may not adhere to long-term prescription regimens. Those who are Muslims believe in individual responsibility for obtaining medical care but may ultimately believe that recovery from illness is in the hands of God.

In addition to their physical modesty, Arab Muslims may be easily embarrassed by personal questions.

Arab Muslims practice and expect high standards of modesty. Much attention has been paid to women's modesty practices, especially as they relate to the wearing of the head scarf, the *hijab*. To be without this covering may cause an Arab woman discomfort. In addition to their physical modesty, Arab Muslims may be easily embarrassed by personal questions. In some cases, their reluctance to disclose private information can affect the efficacy of the clinical encounter. Gynecologic services for Arab women should be provided by a woman clinician, if possible. In some situations, an Arab woman may decline to be examined by a male clinician, in which case the use of verbal descriptions of the ailment may be required for a diagnosis, without a physical examination.

Cleanliness is another important aspect of Islamic tradition. Rules for cleanliness include avoiding things that are considered unclean, such as urine, stool, blood, semen, corpses, pigs, dogs, and alcohol. Prayers occur five times a day and are preceded by bodily cleaning. In addition, personal hygiene practices are undertaken by those who have just used the toilet or engaged in sexual relations.

"Good families" traditionally are considered capable of handling any health crisis, and older Arab Americans may be hesitant to accept help from outsiders, including professionals. Furthermore, mental health problems may be particularly embarrassing to families and may be hidden and not discussed with professionals. Family histories of genetic conditions and illnesses (such as mental illness, retardation, blood disorders, reproductive issues, and chronic illness) may be considered secrets, and the family may wish to protect the lineage by keeping them quiet.

Traditionally, the young adult offspring's chances of marriage are believed to be affected if family medical secrets are disclosed.

Although a minute percentage of the Arab American population (as well as a minute percentage of persons from all majority and minority American cultural groups) may hold extreme beliefs, negative and inaccurate stereotypes about Arab Americans include images of religious fanaticism and suspected membership in terrorist organizations. In addition, Arab women are often viewed as oppressed, abused, or maltreated. To provide the best health care possible to Arab American elders, the astute clinician will make every effort to avoid such stereotypical thinking.

Approaches to Decision Making

Males in the Arab American family may be considered to have more authority with regard to medical decisions than females. It is advisable to ask older Arab American patients early in the clinical association if they prefer to make their own health decisions or if they would prefer to involve or defer to others in the decision-making process. An elderly Arab patient may also wish to have family members present during clinician visits. In such instances, the family should be perceived as a help rather than a hindrance to the clinical encounter.

> *Males in the Arab American family may be considered to have more authority with regard to medical decisions than females.*

Disclosure and Consent

In Arab countries, patients are typically told only the good news about their diagnosis. Doctors may wish to work closely with Arab patients and designated family members when there is a terminal or otherwise serious diagnosis, in order to conform to traditional expectations. It is advisable to explore each patient's preferences regarding disclosure of serious clinical findings early in the clinical association and to reconfirm these wishes at intervals.

In traditional Arab culture, the senior male member of the family is considered the person to give consent for medical procedures and surgeries. Again, the skillful clinician will discuss

> *In Arab countries, patients are typically told only the good news about their diagnosis.*

each individual elder's preferences and reconfirm his or her wishes regarding consent for health care near the beginning of the clinician-patient relationship.

Gender Issues

In traditional Arab societies, the male is responsible for the matters outside the household, while women are considered to be in charge of household activities and child rearing. These ideals are changing among younger cohorts of Arab Americans, especially as women have been found in increasing numbers in the labor force. However, for older adults, the man may still be seen as the person with authority to make decisions—including medical directives. In the most traditional families, men are expected to act in ways that would be consistent with protecting the women of the family with regard to decision making, modesty, privacy, and virginity. Especially among Muslims, the family may have gender-based expectations, where a family may appoint a male member to be the person responsible for the patient's proper care in the health care system. Confirmation of the individual older woman's preferences regarding her own role is essential to the success of the clinical encounter.

Middle Eastern women are often viewed in North America as being gravely oppressed by men. The women's practice of covering their bodies is considered to be evidence of that oppression. However, for many Muslim women, the idea that a woman would expose her body as is done in Western culture is itself considered oppressive and potentially exploitive.

Women in Arab and Muslim families are often highly respected within the household, especially once they have become mothers and grandmothers. Children are raised with a strong obligation to care for aging parents and respect their advice. However, recent research suggests that economic and societal pressures have decreased the time devoted to older parents. Some of this is attributed to the need for adult daughters and daughters-in-law to join the workforce, limiting their ability to spend time in caregiving roles.

End-of-Life Decision Making and Care Intensity

Older Arab Americans with disabling health conditions may at some point need care in a health facility, but cultural norms would encourage the family to exhaust all other available options first. Those with language difficulties may not be able to communicate with nurses and other staff members in a residence facility, causing extreme isolation and confusion. There may also be other issues for Muslims, such as the lack of availability of halal meats and religious supports in the institutional setting. Many older persons living in a facility may feel trapped in an inadequate environment.

After death, family members may have specific wishes regarding what is to be done with the patient's body.

Arabs often believe that death is determined by God's will, but they are not opposed to seeking medical treatment. After death, family members may have specific wishes regarding what is to be done with the patient's body. Traditional customs have the family members involved in a ceremonial washing of the body, and it may also involve wrapping the loved one's body in sheets. Muslim customs prefer immediate burial, so delays in releasing the remains of a loved one to the family should be avoided if possible.

Sonia Salari, PhD
Hashim Balubaid, MD

CASE STUDY **1**	**Accepting the Will of God**

Objectives
1. Understand the cultural aspects of Arab American women's attitudes toward health care workers.
2. Realize how much American Muslims believe in God.
3. Emphasize the degree of trust in the medical profession among Arab Americans.

Sara is a 75-year-old Muslim who was born in Syria. After the death of her husband, she came to the United States 4 years ago to live with her children (two sons and one daughter). She has been living with her eldest son Mustafa since her arrival. Mustafa is a clinical engineer who is married and has two daughters. Over the past year, the family has noticed that Sara has lost weight; her appetite has decreased and she has become less energetic.

You are male and a new internist to Los Angeles, and you have received this new referral from a family physician. The reason for the referral is to assess Sara regarding her weight loss, poor appetite, and anemia to exclude malignancy. The referring physician also mentioned to you that Sara is a Muslim and speaks little English. Coming through the door, you see an elderly lady wearing a scarf on her head, accompanied by two family members: son Mustafa and the daughter Salwa. You greet Sara by trying to shake her hand, but she refuses to do so. The son then immediately shakes your hand, and he introduces his mother and sister to you. Several thoughts come to your mind: that Sara is probably not happy to see you, or that she may be depressed. You ask Mustafa if he will be the interpreter during the interview, and he readily agrees.

Question:
1. What difference will it make to a physician's thoughts and approach if he is aware that female Muslims prefer not to shake hands with males as part of their culture and religion, and that their preference is not a matter of disrespect?

During the interview you find that Sara is very cooperative and has a good sense of humor. By the end of the interview, you have learned that she has a poor appetite and low energy and that she has lost 30 pounds over the past year. Also, you have learned of a strong family history of colon cancer. You explain to Sara that she needs to be admitted to the hospital for a colonoscopy and other necessary investigations.

At the end of the hospital work-up, Sara is found to have iron-deficiency anemia and hypoalbuminemia. The colonoscopy reveals a moderate-sized mass in the ascending colon, and a biopsy reveals adenocarcinoma. A computed tomography scan report tells you that Sara has distant metastasis to the liver, pancreas, and regional lymph nodes, with questionable lung metastasis. You review and discuss these results with the oncology team, and the decision is made that Sara is not a candidate for intervention, but rather that she will receive full supportive care.

As you explain these results to Mustafa, you notice that he becomes anxious and worried; he asks you if there is any way to cure his mother's cancer. Your answer is that unfortunately, there is none, but you reassure him that she will receive supportive care so as to be as comfortable as possible. He acknowledges that there is no cure for her cancer and says that he believes this is God's will. He thanks you for what you have done for his mother. You then ask him about the best way to communicate this information to his mother and the rest of the family. He explains that he will tell the rest of family his way. He also requests that you meet with his mother and the rest of the family tomorrow to discuss the results.

The next day you go to Sara's hospital room and find Sara and Mustafa with his brother and his sister. Mustafa translates to his mother everything that you say. When you finish, Sara thanks you and adds, "I am sure this is my God's will, and thank you God for everything." She asks that she be able to go home, and her family agrees with that request.

You send her home with a referral for hospice care as well as home-health care for home support. Four months later you hear from Mustafa that Sara has passed away peacefully. You learn that the family chose not to use the hospice option or home-health care, preferring instead to take care of Sara themselves. Her adult children, Mustafa explains, believe that it has been their responsibility to take care of their mother themselves, without the use of an unfamiliar hospice team or home-health aide. The use of such formal services, he adds, would have been a sign of the family's shortcoming and an embarrassment.

Questions:
1. How does the involvement of family members insulate the patient in the medical experience?
2. What could be done for patients in Sara's situation who have fewer available family members?
3. How might immigration status limit the support that is available to Arab American elders?

CASE STUDY **2** | **Assessing Comfort with Intervention**

Objectives

1. Show how Arab American families are protective with regard to a history of mental illness.
2. Show the strength of the relationship among Arab American families.
3. Understand some of the cultural and religious beliefs and values behind the avoidance of care facilities for Arab American elders.

Mr. Ali is a 79-year-old man who lives with his wife Jameela in their own home. Mr. Ali was born in Yemen and came to Detroit in 1985. He has one son (Majid) and two daughters (Fatima and Aishah), and all of them live in the same city. The eldest, his son Majid, resides with him in the same house, along with his wife and two children.

Mr. Ali used to work in his own restaurant, but Majid has been taking care of the business for the past 6 years. Mr. Ali is known to have borderline hypertension that does not require treatment, and he also has osteoarthritis of both knees and chronic lower back pain, which all together slightly limit his mobility. His wife and son Majid are his main caregivers.

One night Mr. Ali falls in the bathroom, a fall that results in severe left hip pain. The family immediately takes him to the emergency department, where he is found to have a left hip fracture. He is admitted to the orthopedic floor. The next morning the patient has uneventful surgery for his fracture. Day one postoperatively, the patient is delirious and slightly agitated.

You are the geriatrician on call, and you are asked to see Mr. Ali. The patient is drowsy and disoriented. The nurse tells you that the patient is hallucinating. You introduce yourself to his wife and son, who have just arrived in the room. You ask the family about his baseline cognitive state or if he has had confusion before. The son denies that. Then you ask about his short-term memory; both respond in the affirmative, but the son mentions that it is "expected for his age." Now you inquire about his history of behavioral characteristics, personality changes, and previous hallucinations. The son looks at his mother and then replies that there were a few things, again remarking that all are expected for his age.

Question:

1. What would be the best approach to obtaining a mental health history in an Arab American family?

You repeat your question regarding the patient's behavioral and personality changes and hallucinations, and you reassure the family about confidentiality and the importance of this information. Both of the caregivers start to give you more detailed information. By the end of the interview, you have learned that Mr. Ali has had a short-term memory problem for 4 years, with gradual onset. Over the past year, he has begun to have visual hallucinations and disturbed sleeping, both of which sometimes disturb his wife greatly. Also you learn that his level of consciousness has fluctuated on two occasions during the past year.

Your initial work-up includes complete blood cell count, electrolytes, kidney function, calcium, TSH, serum B_{12}, and folic acid levels; they are all normal. Also, his electrocardiogram and troponin I are normal. A computed tomography scan of the brain reveals mild to moderate cortical atrophy. There are no infarctions or hemorrhages.

With adequate hydration and good pain control, the delirium clears up, and by day three postoperatively Mr. Ali is back to his baseline as described by the family. He is alert but slightly disoriented to the place. He scores 20 out of 30 in the Mini–Mental State Examination, with poor visuospatial skills. You explain to the patient and his family that Mr. Ali has dementia, likely of mixed type (Lewy body dementia and Alzheimer's disease), and that this is not a normal part of aging. You also explain to them that there is a medication that can be helpful in this condition.

The family members are very happy with this good news and agree to the treatment. You also explain to the family that because Mr. Ali's mobility was slightly limited before the fracture, he now needs a prolonged rehabilitation program to recover his baseline functional status. You therefore ask about the possibility of transferring Mr. Ali to a rehabilitative care facility to reduce the burden on the family. Mr. Ali and his wife both refuse. His son explains that his father will not be happy there for traditional, cultural, and religious reasons.

Question:
1. How could the physician help the patient and the family without placing the patient in a rehabilitation facility?

Mr. Ali stays in the hospital for 4 weeks. During that period, you initiate rivastigmine. The patient also follows a good rehabilitation program. Nursing records show that the patient has established a good sleeping pattern and has suffered minimal hallucination. By the time of discharge from the hospital to return home, Mr. Ali requires minimal one-person assistance. You arrange for an outpatient physiotherapy program, a referral for home-health care, and instructions to follow up with you in 6 weeks.

References

Atallah R. Voices of the Arab communities. Available at: http:ethnomed.org/ethnomed/voices/arab.html (accessed November 2005).

Fakhouri H. Growing old in an Arab American family. In: Olson LK, ed. *Age Through Ethnic Lenses: Caring for the Elderly in a Multicultural Society*. Lanham, MD: Roman & Littlefield; 2001:160–170.

Gallaher T. Changing family structures affect health care among elderly Arabs and Arab Americans in Detroit area, according to UM–Dearborn study. Press release University of Michigan–Dearborn, May 18, 2004. Available at: www.umd.umich.edu/univ/ur/press_release/may04/agingstudy_pr.html (accessed November 2005).

Hassoun R. Arab-American health and the process of coming to America: lessons from the metropolitan Detroit area. In: Suleiman MW, ed. *Arabs in America: Building a New Future*. Philadelphia: Temple University Press; 1999:157–176.

Kulwicki A. Health issues among Arab Muslim families. In: Aswad BC, Bilge B, eds. *Family and Gender Among American Muslims: Issues Facing Middle Eastern Immigrants and Their Descendants*. Philadelphia: Temple University Press; 1996:187–207.

Salari S. Aging in the United States. In: Joseph S, ed. *Encyclopedia of Women in Islamic Cultures*. Netherlands: Brill Publishers, 2006;3:14–16.

Salari S. Invisible in aging research: Arab Americans, Middle Eastern immigrants, and Muslims in the United States. *Gerontologist* 2002;42(5): 580–588.

Samhan H. Arab Americans. Available at: www.aaiusa.org/definition.htm (accessed December 2005).

Sengstock MC. Care of the elderly among Muslim families. In: Aswad BC and Bilge B, eds. *Family and Gender Among American Muslims: Issues Facing Middle Eastern Immigrants and Their Descendants*. Philadelphia: Temple University Press; 1996:271–297.

Suleiman MW. Introduction: The Arab immigrant experience. In: Suleiman MW, ed. *Arabs in America: Building a New Future*. Philadelphia: Temple University Press; 1999:1–21.

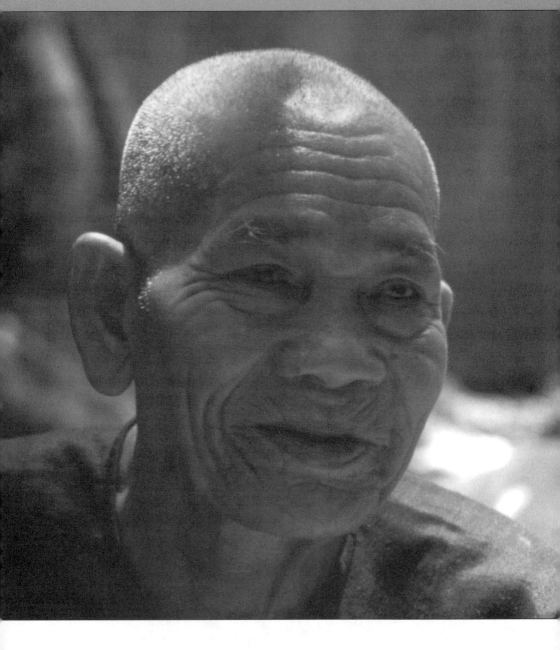

CHAPTER 3

Older Cambodian Americans

Doorway Thoughts

The large majority of Cambodians migrated to North America between 1979 and 1986. The 2000 U.S. Census counted 206,052 Cambodian Americans, approximately 12.2 percent (25,138) of them aged 50 years or older. The Cambodian American population is a more youthful population than other more established minority populations in the United States, including Japanese Americans and Chinese Americans. The 2000 U.S. Census also revealed that Cambodian Americans are poorer than most other Americans; the only ethnic populations in California to have per capita incomes below $10,000 were Hmong Americans, Cambodian Americans, and Laotian Americans. In California, 40 percent of Cambodian immigrants, 32.2 percent of Laotians, and more than half of all Hmong live in poverty.

The Cambodian American population is a more youthful population than other more established minority populations in the United States.

Older Cambodian Americans are a diverse group with respect to education, health and mental health status, impact of migration history, degree of acculturation, and availability of family and local community supports. Organizations serving Southeast Asians in the United States report that barriers to service access for elders include scarcity of language interpreters, cultural consultation, and readily available transportation. In addition, as a result of previous experience abroad, Southeast Asian American elders may fear contact with governmental agencies designed to assist them.

Preferred Cultural Terms

Refugees and immigrants from Cambodia are the Khmer (the most populous ethnic Cambodian group), the Cham (a Muslim minority group), and the Khmer Loeu (or highlander Khmer).

Formality of Address

In formal settings, Cambodian elders may be addressed as Mr. or Mrs. Mony (given name) or Mony Keo (given name and family name). It is rare and impolite to use the family name by itself because use of only the family name refers to a person's father, grandfather, or ancestor, rather than to that specific person. Across informal situations, Cambodians may refer to nonrelatives by endearing family relative names to show deference and respect to someone more senior. For example, they might call an older man *Ta* (grandfather), *Po* (uncle), or *Bang* (brother), or an older woman *Yeay* (grandmother), *Ming* (aunt), or *Bang Srey* (sister). An optimal and culturally competent strategy is to use the formal address until the clinician can determine the preferred name that a Cambodian elder would like used. With increased familiarity and development of the relationship with the Cambodian elder, this degree of formality may not be necessary.

> *It is rare and impolite to use the family name by itself because use of only the family name refers to a person's father, grandfather, or ancestor, rather than to that specific person.*

Language and Literacy

Three quarters of Cambodian elders speak English not well or not at all. Although data regarding their educational status are scarce, it is probable that the majority of Cambodian elders come from rural backgrounds and have little formal education. By implication, the majority of Cambodian elders may have a limited level of literacy both in their own Khmer language (reading and writing) and in English. Agencies serving this population consider translation and interpretation services to be an important factor in making social, mental health, and health services available to Cambodian elders and ensuring their effectiveness.

Respectful Nonverbal Communication

Cambodians greet each other by placing their hands, palms together (*som pas*), with a slight bow and a verbal greeting (*chum reap sur*). Variations in the traditional greeting reflect the degree of respect being shown to the other person. The higher the hands and lower the bow, the more respect is being displayed. A lack of reciprocity in *som pas* greeting between traditional Cambodians would be viewed as insulting. Steady eye contact is not considered respectful, especially when interacting with someone older than oneself or someone considered a superior. The head is considered the most important part of the body because it is the location of a person's spirit. Therefore, it is considered inappropriate to touch an individual's head. Bowing slightly from the waist while walking in front of someone is considered a sign of respect. (For a more detailed review of Cambodian culture, see the EthnoMed Web site, which contains culture and health information by Harborview Medical Center in Seattle, Washington.)

> *Steady eye contact is not considered respectful, especially when interacting with someone older than oneself or someone considered a superior.*

History of Traumatic Experiences

The Cambodian population was terrorized between 1975 and 1979 by the genocidal reign of the Khmer Rouge movement and dictator Pol Pot. An estimated 1.5 million Cambodians, or approximately 20 percent of the total Cambodian population, were killed by execution, disease, or starvation, often in brutal labor camps, at the hands of this regime. According to numerous sources, the Khmer Rouge government relocated 2.5 million city dwellers to rural Cambodia, separated children from parents and spouses from one another, executed a vast number of professionals and individuals educated in the northern hemisphere, and targeted minority groups such as the Cham for total extermination. Such policies resulted in rapid disruption of longstanding traditional Cambodian culture, society, and governance. Refugees and survivors often languished in refugee camps or returned home to find very little remaining. Cambodians who fled their country during this period experienced extreme losses: of family members, of their culture and way of life, and of their social support systems. As a result, many Cambodian American elders who were living in Cambodia at the time of the genocide have had very traumatizing experiences that may have affected both their mental and physical well-being over many years. The long-term consequences of these events for many Cambodian American elders are discussed in the following section on culture-specific health risks.

Immigration Status

The majority of Cambodian elders came as refugees to the United States from 1979 to 1986; the total number was approximately 122,000. The first wave of Cambodian refugees (5700 people) had strong connections with the U.S. government and were customarily Western-educated, with English- or French-speaking abilities. Most fled from the Khmer Rouge from 1975 to 1979. According to the 2000 U.S. Census, Cambodian Americans were located in California (85,559), Massachusetts (22,886), Washington (16,630), Pennsylvania (10,207), Texas (8225), and Minnesota (6533). About 45.7 percent of Cambodians have become U.S. citizens. Approximately 32 percent of Cambodians are linguistically isolated, and an estimated 82 percent of Cambodian elders have poor English skills (i.e., speaking English not well or not at all). In 1999, the median family income among Cambodian Americans was $35,434, and 29 percent were living below the poverty level. In California, approximately 25 percent of Cambodian American elders live in poverty; a similar percentage is estimated to receive fewer Social Security benefits than they are eligible for.

Degree of Acculturation

Interpretation and translation services have been identified as a critical need wherever Cambodian American elders seek health services.

The majority of Cambodian American elders live in traditional ways and are less acculturated than their younger family members; this may be especially true of the elders who came to the United States after 1979. One indicator of acculturation may be proficiency in English. Because so few Cambodian American elders are proficient in English, interpretation and translation services have been identified as a critical need wherever they seek health services. The astute clinician will ask the older Cambodian American patient early in the clinical relationship about his or her preferences with regard to primary language, comfort levels regarding Western medicine, use of traditional remedies, and truth telling and health decision making. These topics are discussed in the relevant sections to follow.

Tradition and Health Beliefs

Prior to 1975, each Cambodian family owned its own rice paddy and grew its own vegetables. White rice was a staple of the diet, usually accompanied by fish or meat, vegetables, and fruits. Sweets were a rare addition in the traditional Cambodian diet. Families maintained adequate nutrition and health by growing their own food or exchanging food and goods with other village members.

Traditional Cambodians believe that illness is caused by spirit possession, evil spells cast by other people, mistakes in performance of rituals over the life cycle, or neglect of rituals. Cambodians have traditionally treated their own illnesses and illnesses of family members without the intervention of outside parties. This behavior developed in response to the scarcity of physicians and hospitals in Cambodia and the high costs of Western medical care. In traditional Cambodian practices, illness is conceived as an imbalance of hot and cold elements in the body. Herbal remedies, dermal techniques (e.g., coin rubbing or pinching), special foods, and rituals are all used to restore the balance of these elements and thereby to restore health. If the illness does not respond to the home remedies, then a *khru khmer* (traditional healer) or health practitioner is seen.

Emotional disturbance may be attributed to possession by malicious spirits, to bad karma acquired through misdeeds in past lives, or to bad luck in familial inheritance. As a result, those experiencing emotional difficulties or mental illness traditionally may be hidden from public view, in the belief that they bring shame to the family. As a result, when a person of Cambodian descent is having mental health difficulties, the individual or family members may report physical symptoms rather than acknowledge difficulties with emotional causes.

A common complaint among Cambodians is wind illness (*khyol*), having wind (*kerd khyol*), or catching the wind (*khyol chab*), which is comparable to feeling ill or having a sickness or fever. The wind illness is believed to be caused by imbalance in the body that is caused by

- overwork, lack of food or sleep, and exposure to diverse weather (hot to cold to rain);
- illness from a common cold, diabetes mellitus, or hypertension; or
- imbalance specifically of the four human elements (wind, water, earth, and fire).

Such traditional Cambodian health beliefs are based upon Chinese medicine.

When Western medicine is used, older Cambodian American are likely to expect to receive medications to treat the illness; if medications are not forthcoming, the Cambodian elder may "doctor shop" until medications are finally prescribed.

When Western medicine is used, older Cambodian Americans are likely to expect to receive medications to treat the illness; if medications are not forthcoming, the Cambodian elder may "doctor shop" until medications are finally prescribed. Traditionally, medications are taken until the individual feels better and then are discontinued. In addition, older Cambodian Americans may expect medications to take effect quickly, and they may also adjust medication doses downward in the belief that Western remedies are "too strong." The skillful clinician working with older Cambodian patients may wish to take extra care in explaining medication regimens and negotiating a therapeutic plan where drugs are involved.

Culture-Specific Health Risks

Although there is little national data on the health of older Cambodian Americans, the Centers for Disease Control and Prevention has examined the health status of 1026 Cambodians living in Lowell, Massachusetts, finding some disparities between the health of Cambodians and that of other Asian Americans and major disparities between the health of Cambodian Americans and that of the general U.S. population. Cambodians were found to be three times more likely to report not visiting a doctor because of high costs. Over half of the Cambodian American men smoked (50.4%), and the Cambodian American women smoked (10.9%) more than other Asian American women. The Cambodians were less likely than the white population to eat five servings of fruits and vegetables daily (16.4%) and less likely to have been screened for serum cholesterol (47.7%). The

Cambodian American women were less likely to have had a Pap test (64.2%). Rates of uptake for pneumococcal vaccine (18.8%) and screening mammography rates were also lower than in the white population.

The self-reports of chronic disease rates are lower among Cambodian Americans, but there are indications that ill health in this population may be underreported. For example, the Asian Americans in Lowell who were aged 45 years and older (the majority of whom were Cambodian in this sample) were dying from diabetes mellitus at higher rates than the general population in Massachusetts. Cambodians in California have been found to have four times the rate of stroke of the white population (107 versus 28 per 100,000) and higher cardiovascular mortality. Prevalence of chronic hepatitis B infection is high among Cambodian Americans born in Cambodia, and as a result, incidence rates of liver cancer are higher for Cambodian American men than for the general population. Chewing betel nut by middle-aged and elderly Cambodian women increases the risk of their developing cancers of the mouth.

The Cambodian genocide of the 1970s is considered by social scientists to be one of the human rights catastrophes of the 20th century; the full impact of the social conditions associated with the genocide on the health of Cambodian survivors is not fully understood. Individuals who remained in Cambodia from 1970 through 1980 are estimated to have experienced 8 to 16 major traumatic experiences each. During these years, Cambodians of all ages were subjected to long periods of combat conditions, malnutrition and starvation, slave labor, imprisonment, and physical and psychological torture. Throughout Khmer Rouge years, Cambodians are likely to have suffered illness and injury without benefit of health services. Everyone living in Cambodia at that time was witness to human rights atrocities, including but not limited to executions, massacres, and concentration camp-like conditions. Countless Cambodians lost some or all of their family members as well as their homes and communities. Those who emigrated during or after the genocide also lost much of their traditional way of life.

The Cambodian genocide of the 1970s is considered by social scientists to be one of the human rights catastrophes of the 20th century.

The long-term starvation and malnutrition experienced during those years put individuals at higher risk for organ-system insufficiency, including cardiac muscle damage, mitral valve prolapse, changes in bone composition, neurologic damage, and vision and hearing impairments.

Khmer "weak heart" syndrome (*khsaoy beh daung*), or death from heart palpitations triggered by anger, noise, worry, odor, or exercise, puts some Cambodians at higher risk than the general public for sudden cardiac arrest. Survivors of the Cambodian genocide are also at higher risk for neurologic and mental health sequelae, including depression, posttraumatic stress disorder, and occult brain insults. Of note, rates of alcohol abuse, homicide, and assault are also higher in the Cambodian American community than in the general population.

Handelman and Yeo found that sadness from obsessive thinking about the loss of family members or traumatic events in the killing fields may be an underlying framework for many illnesses experienced by Cambodian American genocide survivors. This condition (*pruit chit* or *kiit charaen*) also produces severe headaches with dizziness. Drinnan and Marmor found that Cambodians may present with conversion reactions manifesting as functional visual loss; this syndrome may be a culturally appropriate expression of trauma resulting from genocide-related experiences. The strong interrelationship between emotional trauma and experience of physical illness illustrates the strong holistic concept of health among Cambodians Americans. Emotional distress may be reported in terms of physical symptoms, and vice versa. In working with older Cambodian Americans, the astute clinician will be mindful of this interrelationship and gently explore issues of both of emotional and physical well-being when an elder's reported symptoms do not readily lead to a diagnosis.

In one study, services identified as having the highest priority for Cambodian elders living in California include interpretation and translation (46%), culturally appropriate meals-on-wheels and food distribution (37%), advocacy (28%), citizenship counseling (26%), health education (22%), health services (22%), and mental health services (20%). Other services needed are transportation (28%), housing (28%), recreation and traveling

(22%), and outreach, counseling, and support groups (20%). The researchers concluded that such services need to be incorporated into a menu of services provided by mutual aid societies and faith-based organizations who are already serving the Cambodian population.

An innovative program in Cambodia indicated that social support groups may facilitate healing from trauma. Although Cambodian trauma victims may resist discussing their traumatic experiences and the development of support groups may be a slow process, it is believed that such groups may advance significantly the mental health of older Cambodians.

Approaches to Decision Making

Cambodian elders are an integral part of Cambodian families. The vast majority of Cambodian elders live with an adult child or in a variety of other living arrangements among family members. By inference, the culturally sensitive clinician will establish, early in the clinical relationship, a Cambodian elder's preferences for inclusion, or not, of family members in making major health decisions.

Even though some Cambodians have adopted the Christian religions of their sponsors from refugee camps, the principles of Theravada Buddhism permeate the Cambodian worldview. Traditional Cambodian and Buddhist values of selflessness, cooperation, and respect, as well as the goal of upholding the family's reputation or "face," commonly guide traditional Cambodian elders and their families to make decisions together. With acculturation, role reversals may take place, with a shift toward greater status of English-speaking and younger family members.

Traditional Cambodian and Buddhist values of selflessness, cooperation, and respect, as well as the goal of upholding the family's reputation or "face," commonly guide traditional Cambodian elders and their families to make decisions together.

Cambodians' cultural and experiential history may color their choices when making health decisions. Cultural and historical experiences, especially those occurring during the genocide or in refugee camps, may remain undiscussed and may create significant barriers to communication between patients and clinicians. For example, after suffering extreme persecution at the hands of the Khmer Rouge government, Cambodian Americans may feel a global distrust of all governmental agencies, even those in the United States. As a result, Cambodian Americans may not utilize government-sponsored services if they can avoid it. Similarly, social taboos such as discussions of breast health may impede efforts to educate older Cambodian American women with regard to breast self-examination and screening mammography.

Disclosure and Consent

Discussion of the end of life and death and dying traditionally is contained within Cambodian families. As in some other Asian cultures, Cambodian families may seek to shield a family member from knowing about a poor prognosis, because such knowledge may be believed to contribute to ill heath, cause a patient to lose hope, or in fact cause death itself. Customarily, Cambodian Americans may have great faith in the ability of Western medicine to cure disease; as a consequence, there may be substantial reluctance to forgo any treatment.

In traditional Cambodian culture, pain and discomfort are endured stoically.

In traditional Cambodian culture, pain and discomfort are endured stoically. Clinicians working with Cambodian elders may wish to ask about how the patient is experiencing each symptom.

Clinicians are advised to establish a Cambodian American elder's preferences regarding who should receive health information from clinicians, who should make his or her health decisions, and who should give consent for medical procedures, all well in advance of urgent health problems. Particular sensitivity and patience may be required in crafting end-of-life plans for patients or their loved ones because of traditional social proscriptions against speaking about the impending death.

Gender and Social Issues

Equality has traditionally been greater for Cambodian women than for women from some surrounding Asian countries. However, in traditional society, Cambodian women have been expected to respect male authority and privilege, especially in public places.

In many cases, family wealth and status were forfeited during the Cambodian genocide and its aftermath, resulting in a loss of social and financial rank for many Cambodian American elders. The acculturation of younger Cambodian Americans and their children born in the United States may lead to intergenerational tensions, because traditional or linguistically isolated elders wield less influence within families and in society at large than their English-speaking children and grandchildren. It is advisable to remain alert to such possibilities when working with Cambodian American elders, without assuming that this is the case for all families. Should such issues affecting clinical situations arise, respectful inquiry into the gender and social roles in each patient's family is recommended.

Equality has traditionally been greater for Cambodian women than for women from some surrounding Asian countries.

End-of-Life Decision Making and Care Intensity

End-of-life decision making is influenced by health beliefs and beliefs about death and the afterlife. The majority of Cambodians are Buddhist or Christian and adhere to beliefs about karma and reincarnation, with concern for the influence of ancestral spirits. Hospitals may be avoided and critical medical attention may be delayed because of the belief that souls of people who have died in the hospital can disturb or harm the living who visit the hospital.

Hospitals may be avoided and critical medical attention may be delayed because of the belief that souls of people who have died in the hospital can disturb or harm the living who visit the hospital.

Heroic medical interventions such as cardiac resuscitation or being surrounded by strangers while dying may be regarded as a "bad death" by Cambodians. Dying at home may be believed to have the potential to offer more cultural and community support than dying at the hospital. Preparation of the body after death includes washing by family members, putting hands in the prayer positions with candles, placing incense in the hands, and, in some families, inserting a coin in the mouth of the deceased. Cambodians customarily prefer the funeral rite of cremation.

Use of Advance Directives

There is no published information regarding the use of advance directives in the Cambodian American community. As with all intercultural communication issues in health care, it is recommended that discussion of advance directives take place at a time when clinician and patient have had a chance to get to know one another, but if possible well in advance of any health crisis. The culturally astute clinician will approach the subject with diplomacy and tact, taking into account each older Cambodian American patient's wishes regarding disclosure, consent, and decision making. Please refer to the relevant sections in this chapter for information regarding these associated issues.

Barbara W.K. Yee, PhD
Yani Rose Keo, Cambodian elder

CASE STUDY **1**	# Impact of Cambodian Life History and Health Beliefs in a Western Medical Context

Objectives
1. Examine how historical events affect the personal situations of Cambodian elders, influencing their ability to cope with health issues.
2. Examine Cambodian beliefs of disease, dying, and hospitalization.

Mrs. Samnang is a 65-year-old woman who was born in a small village of the northwest province in Cambodia. She has never been to school, and she had an arranged marriage. She has been a housewife and raised ten children, while her husband went to work in the rice field as farmer.

During the war in 1973, her husband was selected to be part of the army for the Republic of Cambodia. In 1975, the country fell to the Communist regime (Pol Pot), and Mrs. Samnang, the children, and her husband were separated by the regime. All the children except the two youngest were taken away from her to work. Her husband was also taken away; he never returned and was likely executed by the Khmer Rouge. Later, she learned that five of her children died of starvation and disease. In 1980, she located two of the children who had been taken, and they were reunited with their mother and two youngest siblings. In late 1982, Mrs. Samnang and her children decided to escape Cambodia, and they walked toward the Cambodian border with Thailand, where they found help in the refugee camp that had been set up by the United Nations High Commission for Refugees. They stayed in the refugee camp for more than 4 years, until one of the voluntary agencies in United States sponsored them and brought them to the United States. Her two older children were unable to attend school because of their ages, and they found work to support the family. The younger 2 children have been treated for psychiatric disorders; over 10 years they have been admitted multiple times for depression and suicidality.

Recently, Mrs. Samnang started to have abdominal pain and vaginal bleeding. Instead of going to a Western doctor, she has been coining herself, and she also prays to get better. She has warned the children not to tell anyone, especially the case worker who visits her regularly. During a home visit, the case worker observes that Mrs. Samnang is weak and pale. On further questioning, Mrs. Samnang admits that she has been bleeding. The case worker strongly encourages Mrs. Samnang to go to the emergency department or to see a doctor.

Question:

1. Why would Mrs. Samnang be resistant to seeking Western medical attention? How might the case worker handle her concerns?

The case worker has long conversations with Mrs. Samnang over a few weeks. She is concerned about the welfare of her two youngest children, who are still struggling with depression. Mrs. Samnang also feels that she has to look after her grandchildren so that her older children can work and support the rest of the family. She finally lets the case worker arrange a family meeting, at which time they assure their mother that they can make alternate arrangements while she goes to the hospital. The case worker and her daughter accompany Mrs. Samnang to the hospital; her daughter asks to be present at all examinations. The case worker asks for female clinicians, because she knows that Cambodian women usually do not allow pelvic examinations by male physicians.

After many tests, the doctors find that Mrs. Samnang has uterine cancer. She asks the case worker to take her to the religious temple to be blessed by the highest priest. During her treatment for cancer, she is given medication to take daily. Mrs. Samnang does not take the prescribed medications and instead buys herbal medication.

Question:

1. How could the health care team manage Mrs. Samnang's nonadherence to her cancer treatment?

Close follow-up is arranged by health professionals and bilingual case workers with the patient and her family members. They explain in great detail the importance and reasons for adherence with medication regimens and follow-up medical visits.

Eventually, though, Mrs. Samnang is admitted to the hospital. She tells the case worker that she would rather die at home than at the hospital or nursing home. She complains that she cannot eat the food that is provided by the hospital. Family members bring comfort foods of rice and soups and arrange for delivery of food from the local Cambodian restaurant. She is still despondent and cries frequently.

Question:

1. Why would Mrs. Samnang continue to want to return home?

Finally, she admits that she is afraid that the spirits of the dead are present at the hospital and that they are a negative energy. She believes that she will die and that being at the hospital means that she will have a "bad death." Some members of the health care team think she requires a psychiatric referral, but after further discussion with the family, they realize that these are culturally appropriate beliefs. At her request,

she is released her from the hospital and follow-up is arranged with visiting nurses.

At home, Mrs. Samnang is happy and even takes the medications
that were prescribed to her by the doctor. Sadly, 4 months later Mrs.
Samnang perishes, leaving her four children and grandchildren.

CASE STUDY **2**	**Posttraumatic Stress Disorder and Holes in the Family**

Objectives
1. Recognize the symptoms of posttraumatic stress disorder in an older Cambodian refugee.
2. Discuss details of Mr. Odom's personal history that influence disease presentation.

Mr. Odom is a 67-year-old man who was born in a small village on the border of Cambodia and Thailand. Mr. Odom was sent by his family to become a monk in his early teens. Later, Mr. Odom became a farmer, a husband, and a father to three children. During the fall of Cambodia in 1975, the family members were separated from each other by the Khmer Rouge. In 1979, when the Vietnamese communists invaded Cambodia, Mr. Odom and his family reunited. In the early 1980s, the family decided to escape Cambodia and planned to walk to Thailand, believing that they could reach the refugee camp there. On the way to Thailand, Mr. Odom's wife and children stepped on a mine and were killed instantly. Mr. Odom continued to walk by himself to the refugee camp, where he succeeded in finding help from the United Nations High Commission for Refugees.

During his 2 years in the refugee camp, Mr. Odom met a fellow refugee; they were married and had a child. Later, they were accepted and sponsored by a voluntary agency and came to the United States. Upon their arrival, Mr. Odom was registered in school to learn English as a second language, along with other refugees. He found a manual labor job at a local warehouse.

After 10 years Mr. Odom lost his job; now he has begun to have headaches and stomach pain. He smokes and drinks heavily. He has had a fall, breaking his hip. After returning home from the hospital, he resumes drinking and will not take his medication. He tells the family not to tell the case worker. However, his wife goes to see the case worker and asks for her help, saying that her husband has started to hallucinate and talk to himself. According to his wife, Mr. Odom sits in the middle of the living room at night and lights tree branches that he has gathered from outside, thinking that he is in Cambodia with his first wife and children. With the help of the case worker, his wife brings him to the hospital. There the physicians exclude any physical causes of the headaches and stomach pain.

Questions:

1. What is the explanation for Mr. Odom's somatic and psychological symptoms?
2. What factors in Mr. Odom's personal history are influencing his behavior and disease presentation?

Mr. Odom is referred to a psychiatrist, and she diagnoses posttraumatic stress disorder and depression. He spends 2 weeks in hospital; the hallucinations improve with medication. At this point, he denies suicidality and insists on returning home. The physician knows that she cannot keep him against his will, and he goes home with a prescription for medications. At home he does not fill the prescription, and instead he asks to be blessed by a Buddhist monk and takes herbal remedies. Unfortunately, a week later Mr. Odom dies in a fire he has set in his living room.

References

Becker G, Beyene Y, Newsom E, et al. Creating continuity through mutual assistance: intergenerational reciprocity in four ethnic groups. *J Gerontol B: Psychol Sci Soc Sci* 2003;58(3):S151–S159.

Cambodian Health Network. Health crisis. Available at: www.cambodian health. org/healthcrisis.asp (accessed September 2005).

Carlson EB, Rosser-Hogan R. Trauma experiences, posttraumatic stress, dissociation and depression in Cambodian refugees. *Am J Psychiatry* 1991;148 (11):1548–1551.

Centers for Disease Control and Prevention. Health status of Cambodians and Vietnamese—selected communities, United States, 2001–2002. *MMWR Morb Mortal Wkly Rep* 2004;53(33):760–765.

Chan, S. Survivors: Cambodian refugees in the United States. Urbana: University of Illinois Press; 2004.

Drinnan MJ, Marmor MF. Functional visual loss in Cambodian refugees: a study of cultural factors in ophthalmology. *Eur J Ophthalmol* 1991;1(3): 115–118.

Handelman L, Yeo G. Using explanatory models to understand chronic symptoms of Cambodian refugees. *Fam Med* 1996;28:271–276.

Hinton D, Hinton S, Um K, et al. The Khmer "weak heart" syndrome: fear of death from palpitations. *Transcult Psychiatry* 2002;39:323–344.

Igasaki P, Niedzwiecki M. *Aging Among Southeast Asian Americans in California: Assessing Strengths and Challenges, Strategizing for the Future.* Washington, DC: Southeast Asia Resource Action Center (SEARAC); 2004.

Keovilay L, Rasbridge L, Kemp C. Culture and the end of life. *J Hospice Palliative Nurs* 2000;2:144–151.

Kinzie JD, Denney D, Riley C, et al. A cross-cultural study of reactivation of posttraumatic stress disorder symptoms: American and Cambodian psychophysiological response to viewing traumatic video scenes. *J Nerv Ment Dis* 1998;186(11):670–676.

Mollica RF, Henderson DC, Tor S. Psychiatric effects of traumatic brain injury events in Cambodian survivors of mass violence. *Br J Psychiatry* 2002;181: 339–347.

Mollica RF, McInnes K, Poole C, et al. Dose-effect relationships of trauma to symptoms of depression and post-traumatic stress disorder among Cambodian survivors of mass violence. *Br J Psychiatry* 1998;173:482–488.

Niedzwiecki M, Yang KY, Earm S. *Southeast Asian American Elders in California: Demographics and Service Priorities Revealed by the 2000 Census and Survey of Mutual Assistance Associations (MAAs) and Faith-Based Organizations (FBOs).* Washington, DC: Southeast Asia Resource Action Center (SEARAC); 2003.

Pachuta DM. Chinese medicine: the law of five elements. In: Sheikh AA, Sheikh KS, eds. *Eastern and Western Approaches to Healing: Ancient Wisdom and Modern Knowledge.* New York: John Wiley & Sons; 1989:64–90.

Reichart PA, Schmidtberg W, Samaranayake LP, et al. Betel quid-associated oral lesions and oral Candida species in a female Cambodian cohort. *J Oral Pathol Med* 2002;31(8):468–472.

Smith-Hefner NJ. *Khmer American: Identity and Moral Education in a Diasporic Community.* Berkeley: University of California Press; 1999.

Southeast Asia Resource Action Center. Refugee arrivals to the U.S. from Southeast Asia, fiscal years 1975–2002. Available at: www.searac.org/refugee_stats_2002.html (accessed September 2005)

van de Put WACM, Eisenbruch M. Internally displaced Cambodians: healing trauma in communities. In: Miller KE, Rasco LM, eds. *The Mental Health of Refugees: Ecological Approaches to Healing and Adaptation.* Mahwah, NJ: Lawrence Erlbaum Associates; 2004:133–159.

Vaughn G, Kiyasu E, McCormick WC. Advance directives preferences among subpopulations of Asian nursing home residents in the Pacific Northwest. *J Am Geriatr Soc* 2000;48(5):554–557.

Yee BWK. Health and health care of Southeast Asian elders: Vietnamese, Cambodian, Hmong and Laotian elders. Ethnic specific modules. Available at: www.stanford.edu/group/ethnoger (accessed September 2005).

Zimmer Z, Kim SK. Living arrangements and socio-demographic conditions of older adults in Cambodia. *J Cross-Cult Gerontol* 2001;16:353–381.

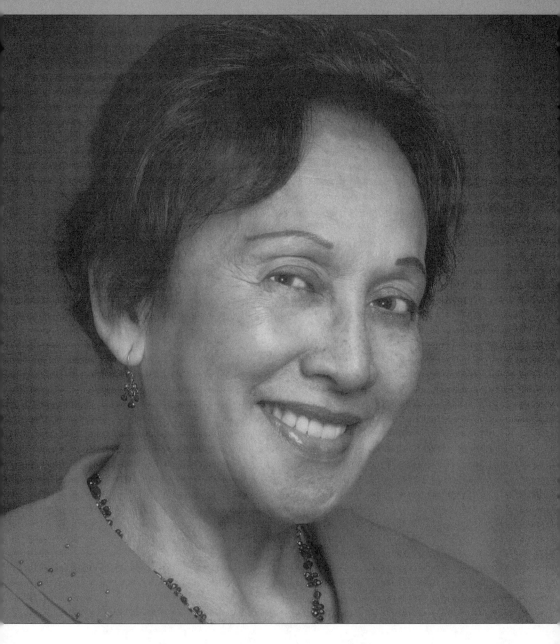

CHAPTER 4

Older Filipino Americans

Doorway Thoughts

Many older Filipinos are part of extended family systems, which include biologic, social, and spiritual ties. Emphasis is placed on interpersonal relations, group harmony, loyalty, respect for elders and authority, and balancing interdependent and dependent functions within this complex support system. Filipino American elders may have a strong preference for talking to a family member, friend, minister, or other trusted person in the elder's inner network before formal health or social service is accessed. Clinicians are advised to become familiar with the patient's informal resources in order to promote prompt care and help the patient avoid social isolation.

Preferred Cultural Terms

In general, the current cohort of elders prefers *Filipino* to designate cultural and ethnic identity. *Filipino American* is acceptable as a formal term; U.S.-born and highly acculturated immigrants use it extensively. *Pilipino* or *Pilipino American* evolved during the civil rights activism of the 1960s. It is considered a symbol of socioeconomic and political autonomy from the historical legacy of colonization. Many community service organizations and student groups have adopted this term. *Pilipino* also refers to the national language of the Philippines.

Pinoy (male) or *pinay* (female) designate gender. Immigrants in the early 1900s, who were mostly men, called each other *pinoy* to symbolize brotherhood. Filipino elders may also use regional terms to give context to their cultural identity. The elder who says "I am Ilocano" (or Tagalog, Cebuano, Bicolano) is self-identifying

Filipino American elders may have a strong preference for talking to a family member, friend, minister, or other trusted person in the elder's inner network before formal health or social service is accessed.

as a native of a specific region in the Philippines, where language and distinct indigenous cultural practices and beliefs differentiate the people from other Filipinos. Terms such as *beterano* (veteran), *Alaskeros* (Filipinos who worked in Alaska), or *sakadas* (plantation contract workers) identify individuals with specific occupational and social histories.

Formality of Address

Filial piety and respect for elders is very strong in Filipino families. The young are taught to use the titles *Lola* (grandmother) and *Lolo* (grandfather) when speaking to or about their elders. The clinician at the first encounter is strongly advised to show respect by initially addressing the older person as Mr., Mrs., or Miss. Including the word *po* in the social greeting, as in "How are you, po?" conveys respect. An adventurous clinician may say "Kumusta po kayo?" The terms *Manang* (female elder) or *Manong* (male elder) plus the first or last name may be used with permission when a degree of comfort in the relationship has been established. When explaining or giving instructions, in order to emphasize a respect for elders, it is advisable to avoid asking the question "Do you understand?" Instead, ask the patient to repeat the information, emphasizing that it is for the clinician's benefit, to ensure that a thorough job has been done.

> *Including the word* po *in the social greeting, as in "How are you, po?" conveys respect.*

Language and Literacy

Pilipino or Tagalog, the national language, is one of eight major Filipino languages (Tagalog, Cebuano or Sebuano, Bikol, Ilocano or Ilokano, Ilonggo or Hiligaynon, Pampango or Pampangan, Pangasinan, and Waray or Samar-Leyte). However, "Taglish," a hybrid of English mixed with Tagalog, is often used in business or social conversation. Although most older Filipinos have basic skills in Tagalog and English, 56 percent of the current cohort of older Filipinos claim that they do not speak English very well. Forty-three percent of those aged 65 and over have less than a ninth-grade education; clinical organizations may wish to develop educational materials accordingly. As more older Filipinos immigrate to join their families, community agencies are reporting a slight increase in the number of elders who are monolingual in one of the Filipino languages. When a medical interpreter is required, it is advisable to frame the service as being necessary to help the clinician provide the appropriate treatment. This approach helps maintain the patient-provider relationship and preserves the older person's self-esteem.

Respectful Nonverbal Communication

Nonverbal communication in the Filipino community is a highly intuitive, contextual process focused on creating and maintaining smooth interpersonal relationships. The older Filipino patient will commonly accept a genuine smile and eye contact with a firm handshake. It is suggested that the clinician greet the patient first when a family member is present. Among highly traditional elders, prolonged eye contact with the clinician is usually avoided as a sign of respect for authority.

Nonverbal communication in the Filipino community is a highly intuitive, contextual process focused on creating and maintaining smooth interpersonal relationships.

Even though young female providers at initial encounters may shake hands with older Filipino men, it may be advisable to refrain from holding a hand to comfort the person unless a well-established clinical relationship and understanding are present. Older women may prefer a female physician. An older Filipino patient may more readily express emotions and concerns with a middle-aged clinician than with a younger one.

Head nodding by a patient has a range of interpretation, one of which is simply being respectful to the speaker without full comprehension of the message. Sitting at eye level with the patient enables the clinician to observe better any head-nodding behavior in the communication process. By giving small amounts of information with brief pauses in between, the clinician will have the opportunity to ask in a gentle manner what a nod of the head means. The clinician might say, "I see you are nodding your head; please tell me what I said that you agree with."

Using simple illustrations or models with explanations and writing instructions in a prescription pad—for example, "walk every day for 30 minutes" and signing it—can convey genuine in-

Using simple illustrations or models with explanations and writing instructions in a prescription pad can convey genuine interest in the elder's welfare.

terest in the elder's welfare. The "prescription" is often treated as an authoritative document that the patient can refer to and use to schedule activities in the household.

History of Immigration

There are documented accounts of the presence of merchant seamen called "Manila men" (i.e., Filipinos) in Alaska and the cities of Los Angeles and New Orleans in the 17th and 18th centuries. Descendants of those who settled in Louisiana are now ninth-generation Americans. More "official" immigration to the United States began in the early 1900s after the Spanish-American War in 1898.

Filipino Americans are the third-largest immigrant population in the United States after the Hispanic-Latino group, and older Filipinos constitute the second-largest Asian American group after Chinese Americans. Though the present cohort of elderly Filipinos is very diverse, it includes predominantly older immigrants who are followers of adult children to help the family. Others have "aged in place" after they immigrated as children and young adults. The latter group is part of the "Philippine brain drain" of the 1960s and those who escaped the Marcos regime.

Filipino Americans are the third-largest immigrant population in the United States after the Hispanic-Latino group.

The most recent arrivals are elderly World War II veterans who were granted U.S. citizenship without veteran's benefits when they immigrated in the late 1990s; they have little social support. Living on Social Security Supplemental Income (SSI), they may be very vulnerable. Many have died while waiting for legislation to restore benefits. The first wave of aging Filipino baby boomers is expected to be even more diverse in historical and demographic characteristics, with a larger proportion of individuals born in the United States.

History of Traumatic Experiences

A large number of the oldest surviving Filipino elders are likely to have experienced blatant discrimination as workers in Hawaiian sugar plantations, California farms, Alaskan fisheries, the U.S. restaurant industry, and domestic service. Their children, who are now the "young-old" Filipinos, grew up with deep awareness of social inequities and intolerance, including inequities in access to and quality of health services. The astute clinician will keep these issues in mind when working with older Filipinos and their families, and will work with the suggestions in this chapter and from other sources to enhance the efficacy of the clinical encounter.

Some older Filipino men may be survivors of the Bataan March in World War II, during which 70,000 American and Filipino prisoners of war were tortured and marched by Imperial Japanese troops over 100 kilometers in extreme heat with little food or water. Only 54,000 prisoners reached the destination prisoner-of-war camp. It was considered one of the major crimes of the war. Survivors of the Bataan March may suffer from a variety of related health consequences, including post-traumatic stress disorder. Clinicians are advised to ask sensitive but direct questions regarding wartime experiences when caring for older Filipino men who may have served with the American military during World War II.

Degree of Acculturation

The contemporary Filipino culture is a unique blend of ancestral cultures (mostly Malayan, Chinese, and Asian Indian) and religious customs (Christian and Muslim), as well as the influences of Spanish and American cultures left behind after colonization ended. Studies have demonstrated a strong preference for Filipino cultural practices and values, particularly with regard to social interactions, accessing resources, and overall lifestyle. However, Filipino elders are commonly resilient culturally and are likely to be able to adapt to North American ways when necessary. Length of residence in the United States may not be the most reliable indicator for acculturation, especially

> *The contemporary Filipino culture is a unique blend of ancestral cultures (mostly Malayan, Chinese, Asian Indian) and religious customs (Christian and Muslim).*

when the patient lives in a multigenerational household. Knowing the elder's English literacy, employment history, occupation, recreational activities, and media preferences may be more helpful in assessing his or her acculturation level. As with all cultural groups, it is important to discuss cultural preferences with each individual patient rather than to rely on generalizations based on cultural assumptions.

Tradition and Health Beliefs

Cultural practices and beliefs about health among older Filipinos are deeply rooted in tradition and religion. For many elders, the numerous influences in Filipino culture have shaped attitudes, behavior, and thinking regarding illness. Filipino elders who have spent the majority of their adult life in the United States may be more accepting of Western biomedical views. More traditional Filipino approaches integrate concepts of illness as being

- a humoral imbalance between "hot" and "cold" in the body system
- divine retribution for sins of omission or commission
- the role of evil spirits or witches exacting punishment for wrongful deeds
- the consequence of such natural events as cold drafts, thunder, lightning, or typhoons

Most Filipino elders use a dual system of health care, blending modern medicine with the traditional practices and principles (supernatural objects and rituals, herbal treatments, and folk medicine). When appropriate, a clinician might ask about the need for spiritual guidance and prayer while health decisions are being made. Some patients and their families may also consult a folk healer. If the clinician knows of this intent, he or she should support the patient's desire to make decisions and ask to share the information in order to reach a comprehensive approach to the treatment plan.

Physicians and other health professionals are customarily accorded high respect and admiration in Filipino culture. At times, this may be a disadvantage because the patient may be reluctant to reveal the use of folk medicine so as not

> *Most Filipino elders use a dual system of health care, blending modern medicine with the traditional practices and principles (supernatural objects and rituals, herbal treatments, and folk medicine).*

to offend the clinician. Filipinos generally accept recommendations for laboratory tests and medical or surgical procedures, but some may insist on getting family members involved in decision making (even those who are back in the Philippines). Health-related cultural beliefs and expectations should be explored with tact and sensitivity so that questions may be clarified and confusion and misunderstanding avoided.

Home Care and Food
Older Filipinos living in the community reside in a variety of types of living arrangements: multigenerational households, shared housing with extended family or friends, senior housing, board-and-care homes, and homeless shelters. It is advisable to include domiciliary information and information on the elder's role and responsibility in the home during the geriatrics assessment. When frailty sets in, family members often depend on their own resources and may be reluctant to access home-care or respite services. Reassurance and encouragement may be necessary to convince elders to seek assistance on a trial basis. A family member from the Philippines may be brought to the United States as a live-in caregiver (*bantay*), or the patient may be taken back to the Philippines, if financially feasible.

To many Filipino elders, food is more than a source of nourishment. Home cooking is a social event; a means to take care of the family's needs and the community; a medium to share family anecdotes, cultural beliefs, and values; and occasionally a way to earn a few dollars. A traditional tropical diet with regional variations from the more than 7000 islands of the Philippine archipelago includes steamed or fried rice served with a dish of small pieces of meat (chicken, pork, beef, seafood) mixed with vegetables, and a dessert of fresh fruit or sweets (rice cake, candied pili nuts). Coconut milk and coconut oil, fish sauce (*bagoong* and *patis*), soy sauce, and tomato sauce are common ingredients. Adapting to current standards of a healthy diet is a gradual process; eating rice, often with every meal, and the use of high-salt seasonings and salt-cured fish are still common practices among Filipinos. Clinicians may need to consider a culturally sensitive multistep approach with psychological support when reduced carbohydrate or salt intake is a part of the treatment plan for a Filipino elder.

Ethnic-Specific Health Risks

Although health data on older Filipino Americans are limited, Filipino elders are considered to be at risk for hypertension, cardiovascular diseases, diabetes mellitus, gout, tuberculosis, hepatitis B, and metabolic problems. There are regional differences in their risk for breast cancer, and Filipino women have the lowest breast cancer survival rate among minorities in the United States, with the exception of African American women. No specific studies on risk factors for various types of dementia have been published; however, vascular dementia may be more common in this population in view of the high prevalence rates of coronary heart disease and hypertension among Filipino Americans.

Filipino women have the lowest breast cancer survival rate among minorities in the United States, with the exception of African American women.

Available studies suggest that the overall prevalence of psychiatric disorders among Filipino Americans is similar to that of other American groups, although the presentations may differ. In general, Filipino Americans present with higher rates of somatic complaints when depressed but have a lower suicide rate (3.5/100,000) than U.S. whites (12.8/100,000). A small but increasing number of pathologic gamblers in the U.S. Filipino community has been reported. Delayed utilization of mental health services may be related to several issues, including but not limited to

- a lack of familiarity with such resources
- a belief that the service is only for those who are "crazy"
- fear of stigma
- preference for first consulting a trusted person
- desire to protect the family from shame and embarrassment
- cost of care

Although Filipino elders suffering from major depression may present with a variety of somatic complaints, the astute clinician will conduct a careful assessment to exclude a local organ system cause for reported symptoms before conducting a psychological assessment or referring the patient to a mental health specialist.

Approaches to Decision Making

Filipino Americans tend to emphasize and value the role of the family in the decision-making process about health care. Families may expect to be involved and may expect to be provided with substantial information regarding treatment plans. The family may include uncles and aunts or godparents who have long-standing and close relationships with the patient. In traditional families, major decisions are commonly delegated to the oldest son or daughter (sometimes, even if they reside outside the United States). At times, decision making may be deferred to another family member or someone in the extended family who is a health care professional or a health care employee. The professional, in particular, may be expected to explain and interpret diagnostic procedures, treatment, or test results, as well as to serve as a liaison between the clinicians and the patient and family.

Filipino Americans tend to emphasize and value the role of the family in the decision-making process about health care.

With increasing acculturation, competent elders may want to have more autonomy and independence in making health care decisions. In planning treatment, it is important to ask the older Filipino American early in the relationship about his or her preferences regarding health care decisions to avoid later difficulties during a health crisis.

Disclosure and Consent

Experts propose four phases of the "awareness of dying" process in patients and families that clinicians may find helpful: closed awareness, suspected awareness, mutual pretense awareness, and open awareness. Some Filipinos elders may initially be at either of the first two phases while the family members process medical information. Eventually, the elder may reach open awareness later in the illness trajectory. Although the traditional Filipino family includes extended kin and friends, the immediate family members often become an "autonomous unit" that receives the information and filters what is discussed with the patient. Reasons often cited include the fear that the truth will cause the patient to lose hope and their need to protect the patient from bad news. In many cases, the elderly patient may have an undisclosed awareness of the illness but choose to remain uninvolved and un-engaged in the decision-making process. From a North American perspective, the behavior may be interpreted as being passive. However, elders may accept family involvement as an opportunity to express filial piety and to reciprocate (*utang na loob*) the caring and nurturing provided when the elder took care of the family.

Unengaged behavior may arise from the elder's belief that one should leave one's fate in God's hands (*bahala na*), while directing efforts to deal with challenges to the best of his or her ability. Suffering may be accepted and endured because it is the will of God. In these situations, it is important from the clinical perspective to confer often with patients regarding pain and discomfort, in order to ensure that optimal symptom management is attained.

> *Suffering may be accepted and endured because it is the will of God.*

Because it is common for older Filipinos to respect a clinician's authority and defer to others in making health decisions, an indirect, gradual approach to disclosing information about diagnosis and prognosis may help patients and their families focus on clinical messages. For example, a skillful clinician may start by saying, "There is information we need to talk about. Would you like us to discuss it at this time, would you prefer to have a family member here with us, or would you prefer for me to discuss the problem directly with one of your family members alone?" Once an approach has been determined, information may be disclosed on a timeline that optimizes understanding and care planning.

Patients have the right to defer to their families in making decisions, but there are growing numbers of more acculturated Filipino elders who prefer to make their own decisions. It is important to verify whether the patient is comfortable with the family's making health care decisions and understands conflicts that may exist among family members. When an individual patient prefers family-based decision making, clinicians may wish to refer to a legal health proxy or, when one is not available, to hold a family conference to identify the family spokesperson who will serve as the surrogate decision maker.

Gender Issues

The traditional Filipino family tends to be matriarchal. Filipino men traditionally are expected to be the providers and keep the family safe and secure. In traditional culture, the women take care of the children, grandchildren, and other family members, and manage and maintain a nurturing household. They actively initiate or participate in making major decisions, with careful attention to the male's role as head of household. With social change and educational opportunities, contemporary Filipino American women now have careers as well.

The traditional Filipino family tends to be matriarchal.

Older women who are highly acculturated may view marriage as a partnership. The interplay between cultural and gender roles may become more complex in a multigenerational household. How variations in attitudes influence the provider-patient relationship and the decision-making process must be assessed and understood for each individual patient. In most families, however, spousal approval and support will most likely be critical in health care decisions and the success of treatment plans.

End-of-Life Decision Making and Care Intensity

Within the community of Filipino elders in the United States, opinions and preferences about care at the end of life will vary widely, and the astute clinician will, of course, assess each individual's preferences. Clinicians are advised to ascertain variations and individual differences early in the illness and to factor this information into discussions with individual Filipino elders about end-of-life issues.

When death in the hospital is anticipated, the family may have a strong preference for same-sex staff to take care of the patient. Family members may also wish to participate in the care. It is advisable to discuss such wishes as early as seems appropriate and to negotiate a care plan that is acceptable to all concerned.

About 90 percent of Filipino Americans are Roman Catholics. Many patients and their families may wish to observe religious rituals (e.g., Sacrament of the Sick) and ceremonies during the dying process and after death. Having religious icons, pictures, or objects in the room may be comforting to patients as well as to their families and caregivers. Prayer sessions may be held in the

Often, members of the extended family and close friends expect to pay their respects to the deceased, a process that may require several hours before the body can be taken to the mortuary.

patient's room by church groups throughout the dying period. The family may wish to perform a ritualistic washing of the body after death. Often, members of the extended family and close friends expect to pay their respects to the deceased, a process that may require several hours before the body can be taken to the mortuary. In many communities, it may not be common for Filipino families to request or give consent to autopsy or organ donation.

Attitudes Toward Advance Directives

Experts recommend that conversations about advance directives include goals of care, values and expectations related to life prolongation, proxy decision making, preference for place of death, and potential benefits of hospice. Comparative studies of Asian American groups indicate that Filipinos are less inclined than other Asian American groups to complete advance directives, have less desire for in-home death and hospice services, and seldom choose a no-code status for the patient. Possible reasons for such preferences may include distrust of the U.S. medicolegal system, longstanding disparities in access to care, conflicts with religious beliefs, and proscriptions about discussing death.

Providers who initiate discussions about advance directives with Filipino elders may face resistance from the patient and family. It may help the process if the clinician starts with the designated family spokesperson to request advice and assistance in opening a discussion about advance directives. Participation of a priest or religious advisor who is known to the patient may be appropriate for some situations. Careful use of words that convey concern and respect are advised in conversations with all elders regarding advance directives and end-of-life decision making.

Melen R. McBride, PhD, RN
Rena Nora, MD
Vyjeyanthi S. Periyakoil, MD

| CASE STUDY **1** | **Parental Love and Isolation** |

Objective
1. Discuss approaches to verbal and nonverbal communication that
   (a) facilitate positive interaction with Filipino American elders and
   (b) value the role of the family in the decision-making process.

Mrs. Aida Dugenio, a 68-year-old woman, is brought to the outpatient clinic by her daughter with presenting problems of chronic headaches, stomach pains, and difficulty in sleeping. Mrs. Dugenio came to the United States 2 years ago after her eldest daughter, a nurse, petitioned for her to come as an immigrant. The patient lives with this daughter, her husband who is an Irish American lawyer, and their 3-year-old girl and 1-year-old son.

Dr. Jones is a middle-aged American who has 5 years' experience in group practice in family medicine in a large metropolitan area. He is well known among Asian and Hispanic patients in the community and many of his referrals are by word of mouth.

Dr. Jones greets Mrs. Dugenio and her daughter and invites them to have a seat across from his desk.

Question:
1. How should Dr. Jones approach communication with Mrs. Dugenio and her daughter in order to facilitate a positive interaction with a Filipino American elder?

Dr. Jones introduces himself, shakes Mrs. Dugenio's hand, and asks how the patient would like to be addressed, to which she replies, "Mrs. Dugenio." The daughter interrupts and explains that they have been to two other doctors, who performed all kinds of laboratory tests and examinations. She has brought copies of the results of the tests, which were all within normal limits. The patient continues to have headaches and stomach pains and has not been eating and sleeping well.

Dr. Jones notices that Mrs. Dugenio seems to be somewhat uneasy. He says, "How are you, po?" The patient smiles and apologizes for "being a problem." She says that she is feeling fine and her daughter just worries too much. Dr. Jones suggests that the daughter wait in the next room and asks the patient if he may proceed with the examination.

While taking her blood pressure and doing the physical examination, Dr. Jones asks her about her husband and the rest of the family. At this point, the patient starts to cry and tells him that her husband passed away 3 years ago. All her five children are grown. She thought it would be a good idea to come to this country because she wanted to be with her grandchildren and to be of help to her daughter. She admits that she has become increasingly lonely for friends and relatives she left behind, but she would not consider going back to her homeland. She feels that a lot of money and effort have already been spent to bring her to this country, and she does not want to "abandon" her daughter and grandchildren. She understands that her daughter works full time as a nurse and her son-in-law has a busy law practice, but she wishes that they had a little more time to take her out on weekends. She says that she is getting a bit too old to take care of the children and gets exhausted by the end of the day. She has difficulty sleeping and wakes up very early in the morning, during which time she gets extremely lonely, experiencing a sense of emptiness and helplessness. She is not expected to do house chores, but she does them to help out. She states that she is not her usual self, and she is afraid that if she does not get better, she will be a burden to the family.

Dr. Jones carefully explains to the daughter and the patient that on the basis of his evaluation, he believes Mrs. Dugenio has clinical depression and that he will prescribe medications that would help her feel better and sleep better.

Questions:

1. How should Dr. Jones carefully and tactfully discuss practical treatment approaches other than medications that would allow the patient to maintain connections with the homeland?
2. How should he try to involve the family in this patient's treatment?

Dr. Jones suggests that Mrs. Dugenio needs to have activities that would prevent her from feeling isolated. He asks her daughter to come up with some solutions to involve her mother and emphasizes that this will prevent her mother from being sick. He suggests that Mrs. Dugenio join the local senior citizen center's Sunshine Club, where other Filipinos get together once a week for various activities. Her daughter agrees and also proposes to enroll the children in a local day-care facility for a half a day, thus giving the patient some free time. She will ask her husband to sign up for cable television to have a regular Filipino television channel at home so that Mrs. Dugenio could keep up with current events, movies, and special programs from back home.

Questions:

1. How can Dr. Jones enhance the patient's cooperation and acceptance about taking the medication?
2. What models could he use to highlight the value and benefits of the medications?

Dr. Jones writes out a prescription for medication and also writes out a "prescription" in simple language for Mrs. Dugenio to keep with her. He writes that she should take her pill every day "for eating and energy" and writes out "Tuesday—Sunshine Club" and "Wednesday—free time." He signs and dates the "prescription."

Mrs. Dugenio returns in 6 weeks and reports that she is feeling much improved and is now attending church with friends she made at the Sunshine Club.

CASE STUDY **2**	A Time to Care: The Whole Is More than the Sum of Its Parts

Objective

1. Discuss special characteristics of the Filipino American family system, including the role of religion, that may influence the decision-making process in health care.

Dr. Cornell is an attending physician in family medicine at a large metropolitan hospital on the West Coast. He admits Mr. Luis Guinto, an 84-year-old Filipino with severe heart failure who is not responding to treatment and has been placed on the critical list. He has no advance directive; his 76-year-old wife is anxious and confused about the prognosis and plan of care. She refuses to sign a no-code request and wants to talk to her son, Lou, who is on the East Coast on a business trip. At a family conference call arranged at the hospital, Mrs. Guinto insists that Lou return home to help her handle the situation. Lou speaks with Dr. Cornell, who explains the patient's medical condition. Subsequently, Lou informs his mother that he will take the first available flight home.

Questions:

1. What cultural factors explain Mrs. Guinto's refusal to sign a no-code order and her insistence on having her son come home?
2. Who should be involved in the family decision making at this time? What other services should Dr. Cornell ask to be involved?

While waiting for Lou, the rest of the family takes turns in keeping vigil. Dr. Cornell contacts pastoral services, and they liaise with the family and a Filipino priest from their parish to give Mr. Guinto a blessing for the sick and to bless the family. When Mrs. Guinto is eventually persuaded to go home and get some rest, she does so after she prays the rosary at her husband's bedside. On the way home with Trining, her youngest daughter with whom the couple lives, she talks about the annual family gathering on Christmas Day and expresses the hope that her husband will be well by then.

The next day, Lou comes to the hospital with his mother; two younger sisters; Mr. Carlos Guinto, the patient's brother; and Amalia, a Philippine-born niece who was adopted by the couple when she was orphaned at age 10. At a family meeting, Mr. Guinto's condition is reviewed and treatment options are explained. These options include the replacement of a malfunctioning heart valve. There is a 50-50 chance of the patient's dying during the procedure, and if he lives through it, the long-term outcome of the surgery is uncertain. Without aggressive treatment, Mr. Guinto may live a few weeks to a few months. If the family refuses surgery, the patient will be moved to a palliative care unit in a few days. During the meeting, Mrs. Guinto is quiet most of the time and lets her son and brother-in-law do the talking. Her daughters, Trining and Amalia, want to know what kind of care their father would receive if he is transferred to another unit.

Lou explains that they need some time to decide what is best for their father and the rest of the family. He indicates that he has a brother in the U.S. Marines who is on active duty, that his father's other siblings are vacationing in the Philippines, and that his mother believes her husband will recover as he did from past crises. A friend is already working on scheduling a family conference call for tomorrow morning. Dr. Cornell reassures him that there is time to consult the rest of the family. He thanks them for their cooperation and expresses his appreciation for the way they support each other. Later that day, he receives a call from the admissions office informing him that the palliative care unit is full.

Questions:
1. What alternate care option might the family propose?
3. How should they be supported?

The following afternoon, Dr. Cornell finds Lou and his sisters in the visitor's lounge. They look tired and the women appear to have been crying. Eventually, Lou informs Dr. Cornell that they want to take Mr. Guinto home and asks what they need to do. He says that his mother and sisters are having a difficult time, but that they want to take care of Mr. Guinto. Dr. Cornell calls the hospice care coordinator and introduces her to the family. He reminds the family that he will still be available to their father for his medical care and thanks them for the opportunity to take care of Mr. Guinto.

References

Araneta MR, Wingard DL, Barrett-Connor E. Type 2 diabetes and metabolic syndrome in Filipina-American women: a high-risk nonobese population. *Diabetes Care* 2002;25(3):494–499.

Braun KL, Nichols R. Death and dying in four Asian American cultures: a descriptive study. *Death Stud* 1997;21(4):327–359.

Braun KL, Onaka AT, Horiuchi BY. Advance directive completion rates and end-of-life preferences in Hawaii. *J Am Geriatr Soc* 2001;49(12):1708–1713.

Braun KL, Tanji V, Heck R. Support for physician-assisted suicide: exploring the impact of ethnicity and attitudes toward planning for death. *Gerontologist* 2001;4(1):51–60.

Doukas DJ, McCullough LB. The values history: the evaluation of the patient's values and advance directives. *J Fam Prac* 1991;32(2):145–153.

Kagawa-Singer M. The cultural context of death rituals and mourning practices. *Onc Nurs Forum* 1998;25(10):1752–1756.

Klatsky AL, Armstrong MA. Cardiovascular risk factors among Asian Americans living in northern California. *Am J Public Health* 1991;81(11):1423–1428.

Kogan S, Blanchette P, Masaki K. Talking to patients about death and dying: improving communication across cultures. In: Braun KL, Pietsch JH, Blanchette PL, eds. *Cultural Issues in End-of-Life Decision Making.* Thousand Oaks, CA: Sage; 2000.

Leong FT, Lau AS. Barriers to providing effective mental health services to Asian Americans. *Ment Health Serv Res* 2001;3(4):201–214.

Llamzon TA. *Handbook of Philippine Language Groups.* Quezon City, Philippines: Published for UNESCO by the Ateneo de Manila University Press; 1978.

McBride M, Morioka-Douglas N, Yeo G, eds. *Aging and Health: Asian and Pacific Islander American Elders.* 2nd ed., Working Paper No. 3. Stanford, CA: Stanford Geriatric Education Center; 1996.

McBride MR, Lewis ID. African American and Asian American elders: an ethnogeriatric perspective. *Ann Rev Nurs Res* 2004;22:161–214.

McBride MR, Parreno H. Filipino families and caregiving. In: Yeo G, Gallagher-Thompson D, eds. *Ethnicity and the Dementias.* Washington, DC: Taylor and Francis; 1996.

McFarland CD. *A Linguistic Atlas of the Philippines.* Tokyo: Study of Languages of Asia & Africa Monograph Series No.15; 1980.

Medina BT. *The Filipino Family: A Text with Selected Readings.* Diliman: University of the Philippines Press; 1991.

Miranda B, McBride M, Spangler Z. Filipino Americans. In: Purnell LD, Paulanka BJ, eds. *Transcultural Health Care: A Culturally Competent Approach.* Philadelphia: F.A. Davis Company; 1998.

Nora R, McBride MR. Health needs of Filipino Americans. *Asian Am Pac Isl J Health* 1996;4(1–3):1–139.

Ryan C, Shaw R, Pliam M, et al. Coronary heart disease in Filipino and Filipino-American patients: prevalence of risk factors and outcomes of treatment. *J Invasive Cardiol* 2000;12(3):134–139.

Tan M. *Usug, Kulam, Pasma: Traditional Concepts of Health and Illness in the Philippines.* Quezon City, Philippines: Alay Kapwa Kilusang Pangkalusugan; 1987.

Tompar-Tiu A, Sustento-Seneriches J. *Depression and Other Mental Health Issues: The Filipino American Experience.* San Francisco: Jossey-Bass Publishers; 1995.

U.S. Department of Health and Human Services, Office of the Surgeon General. *Mental Health: Culture, Race and Ethnicity: A Supplement to Mental Health: A Report of the Surgeon General.* Rockville, MD: Department of Health and Human Services; 2001.

Vaughn G, Kiyasu E, McCormick WC. Advance directive preferences among subpopulations of Asian nursing home residents in the Pacific Northwest. *J Am Geriatr Soc.* 2000;48(5):554–557.

Villanueva V, Lipat A. The Filipino American culture: the need for transcultural knowledge. In: Kelley ML, Fitzsimons VM, eds. *Understanding Cultural Diversity: Culture, Curriculum, and Community in Nursing.* Sudbury, MA: Jones and Bartlett; 2000.

Yeo G, Hikoyeda N, McBride, M, et al. *Cohort Analysis as a Tool in Ethnogeriatrics: Historical Profiles of Elders from Eight Ethnic Populations in the United States.* 2nd ed., Working Paper No. 12. Stanford, CA: Stanford Geriatric Education Center; 1998. See also: www.stanford.edu/group/ethnoger.

CHAPTER 5

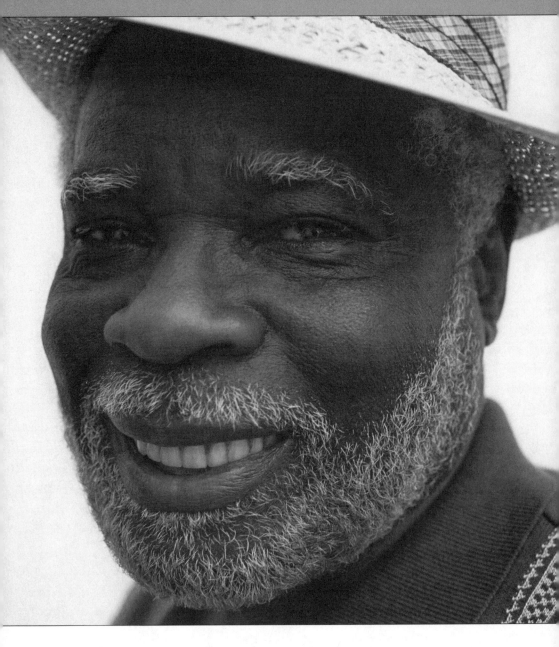

Older Haitian Americans

Doorway Thoughts

The Haitian population in the United States is growing. In the decade between the 1990 U.S. Census and the one in 2000, the number of people reporting Haitian ancestry nearly doubled, rising from nearly 281,000 to approximately 548,000. Haiti has an unusual history, and as a result, many Haitian immigrants to the United States hold a worldview shaped by distinctive religious and historical factors. The Haitian American community, like other ethnic communities in the United States, is diverse, representing all socioeconomic classes. In addition, Haitian culture varies according to whether it is rooted in urban or rural Haiti. The majority of Haitians are Roman Catholics.

In the decade between the 1990 U.S. Census and the one in 2000, the number of people reporting Haitian ancestry nearly doubled, rising from nearly 281,000 to approximately 548,000.

Preferred Cultural Terms

Haitians have analogous genetics and phenotypes to African Americans. Despite their similar appearance to African Americans, Haitian immigrants customarily do not identify with this cultural group. To Haitians, their culture is closely linked to their nationality, and immigrants to the United States will most likely identify themselves as Haitian Americans.

Formality of Address

In Haitian culture, people generally have three names: a first name, a middle name, and a last name. Sometimes the first two names are hyphenated; for example, Marie-Claude. Haitian names are primarily of French origin. Name formats for Haitian women are similar in structure to those used in the United States. When a woman marries, she drops her maiden name and takes her hus-

Eye contact is often avoided in interactions with those in positions of authority and higher social economic status.

band's last name. Traditionally, Haitians are formal and respectful to one another; it is advisable to address Haitians by their title (Mr., Mrs., Miss, or Dr.) until the clinician is able to establish each individual's preferences.

Traditional Haitians commonly use an active tone of voice and direct eye contact when talking with friends. Eye contact is often avoided in interactions with those in positions of authority and higher social economic status.

Language and Literacy

French has always been the language of the educated elite in Haiti, but more than 90 percent of the residents of Haiti speak only Haitian Creole. The origins of Haitian Creole are not fully known, but it is a language in its own right and not merely a form of French. However, Haitian Creole was accepted as an official language only in 1987. Even though only a small percentage of Haitians communicate in French, it is still valued in Haitian culture and is an indicator of social class. Because Creole is viewed as the language of the poor, most Haitians and many Haitian Americans will claim to speak French. A suggestion that someone speaks only Creole, even if that is the case, can be construed as an insult. Because Creole has never been developed as a written language and Haitians have had poor access to schooling, literacy rates among Haitian Americans can be quite low, especially among elders.

Education is highly valued in the Haitian community. It is not uncommon for women to go without food to send their children to school. Many Haitian Americans seek to complete their high school education quickly and will get their high school or equivalency diploma before it is normally required. For Haitians and Haitian Americans, a college degree is a sign of social status and upward mobility.

Respectful Nonverbal Communication

Touch, such as embracing or kissing among persons of the same sex, is accepted in an informal setting. For formal situations, a firm handshake is the proper greeting. Haitians may smile and nod their heads rather than expose their lack of understanding.

In Haiti it is not considered rude to be late to appointments.

Like many cultures outside of North America, in Haiti it is not considered rude to be late to appointments. Because Haitian immigrants may not understand U.S. attitudes regarding time, these patients initially may have difficulty being on time for clinical visits. If punctuality is necessary in a specific clinical setting, it is advisable to stress the need for arriving on or close to the time of the appointment with Haitian American patients. Customarily, patients will try to comply if at all possible.

Acculturation

Factors affecting Haitians' acculturation and assimilation include socioeconomic status, education, religious beliefs and practices, age, reason for migration, and immigration status. Educated and middle-class Haitian immigrants with functional skills in English tend to adopt some aspects of the majority culture more readily than socioeconomically and educationally disadvantaged individuals who have immigrated to escape political persecution or severe poverty. However, it is important not to assume the cultural preferences of older Haitian Americans on the basis of these factors alone. As the clinician gets to know the patient, it is advisable to inquire about specific preferences as they arise during the clinical relationship.

Some Haitians may feel that services offered at clinics or through Medicaid are below acceptable standards because they are free of charge.

Use of North American Health Care Services

In Haiti there is no health insurance, so everyone pays for his or her own health care. Some Haitians may feel that services offered at clinics or through Medicaid are below acceptable standards because they are free of charge. When consulting a biomedical clinician, a Haitian American customarily expects a quick diagnosis, courtesy, the use of a stethoscope, and a prescription. Biomedical care is often used in conjunction with traditional remedies, and the astute clinician will ask older Haitian American patients about *all* of the modes of treatment they are using, acutely or on a regular basis.

Immigration Status

Over the past 40 years, the political and economic climate in Haiti led to a significant increase in the number of Haitians migrating to the United States. Traditionally, Haitians have a deep faith in the future, and this conviction compels some to risk their lives by taking rickety boats to the United States for the sake of their children.

A patient's migration history can sometimes provide information about the patient's social class. The first wave of migration began in 1957 and consisted of professionals who were fleeing the oppressive Duvalier regime. These immigrants were well-educated and obtained visas and work contracts. They were not illegal aliens and had many personal and educational resources to assist them in integrating into American society and resisting some of the racial prejudice prevalent at the time. The second wave, which started in the 1960s and extended through the 1970s, consisted largely of middle-class individuals fleeing economic and political persecution when Duvalier was elected President for Life in 1964. These people also were educated and skilled, and they were accepted and benefited from lenient immigration laws. The last and current group of Haitian immigrants to the United States is made up mainly of members of the lower middle class who are also trying to escape financial and political oppression in Haiti's perpetually unstable political and economic climate. They tend to have limited resources and education. Some arrive in the United States without the necessary immigration documents and have multiple difficulties in obtaining legal status. Unlike prior waves of immigrants, the most recent group has had difficulties with legal status that place a great deal of strain on some Haitian immigrant families, and thereby on their traditional supports and way of life.

Moving elders into care facilities is still a controversial and difficult decision for many Haitian families.

Home Care and Food

In traditional Haitian culture, when elders are no longer able to function independently, they move in with their children. The house is always open to relatives. Older people are addressed by an affectionate title—for example, Aunt, Uncle, Grandma, or Grandpa—even if they are not re-

lated. Elders are highly respected. Their children are expected to care for and provide for
them when self-care becomes a concern. Elders
are family advisors, baby sitters, historians, and
consultants. Relocation to North America may
pose a challenge in traditional family structures

> *When hospitalized, many would rather fast than eat non-Haitian food.*

when children who work have difficulty in caring for their older
parents at home. Moving elders into care facilities is still a controversial and difficult decision for many Haitian families.

During illness, Haitians traditionally like pumpkin soup,
oatmeal, and cream of cornmeal prepared as *akasan*. When hospitalized, many would rather fast than eat non-Haitian food. It is
advisable for clinicians working with hospitalized Haitian American elders to consider allowing family members to bring food
from home.

Tradition and Health Beliefs

The traditional Haitian concept of the real world is that it contains not only what is visible but also what cannot be seen. The
invisible or the spiritual world is made up of good and evil spirits of deceased family members and other supernatural forces.
These spirits can provide information or change a situation. This
tradition extends to Haitians' beliefs about both the natural and
spiritual causes of illness.

Traditional Haitians commonly have a fatalistic but peaceful
view of life. Some believe that fate or spiritual forces are in control of such life events as health problems and death. Haitians
may also believe that they are passive recipients of God's decisions; *si Bondye vle* ("If God wants") is a traditional, common response among Haitians to life's
difficulties. Clinicians are advised to be clear,
honest, and open when assessing each individual's perceptions of the forces that have an influence over life, health, and illness. A nuanced

> *Traditional Haitians commonly have a fatalistic but peaceful view of life.*

understanding of these beliefs is an important factor in building trust and ensuring adherence when working with Haitian
American elders.

Haitian society is stratified, with small upper and middle
classes, and a lower class comprising 85 percent of the popula-

tion. Working-class members commonly acknowledge and practice unconventional modes of therapy, including self-treatments with such modalities as medicines made from plant roots, the much-publicized system of voodoo spiritual practices, and the hot-and-cold regime. This latter system is based on the belief that illness is a result of an imbalance between hot and cold elements in the body. Many Haitians believe a balance of hot and cold foods is necessary to maintain health, and they will treat illness with potent drinks or herbal medicines in the opposite hot or cold class. For example, after performing strenuous activities or any activity that causes increased body heat, it is believed that one should not eat cold food, because this will create an imbalance leading to a condition called *chofret*. The types of traditional Haitian practitioners include herbalists, injectonists, bone setters, and voodoo practitioners. These practitioners are in short supply in the United States, but it is not unusual for families to consult such practitioners and bring herbal preparations back to the United States after visits to Haiti. In some circumstances, Haitian Americans will return to Haiti specifically to be treated by traditional practitioners.

When stressed, as in the case of a life-threatening illness, individuals of all classes will turn to voodoo for help, at the same time practicing their Christian beliefs.

When stressed, as in the case of a life-threatening illness, individuals of all classes will turn to voodoo for help, at the same time practicing their Christian beliefs. Voodoo is a religion of African origin with some contribution from the Taíno Indians who populated the island of Hispaniola (where Haiti is located) before the arrival of European settlers. The primary gods of voodoo, called *loas*, are mostly the spirits of African ancestors. Once Christianity was introduced by the Spaniards to the Taíno Indians and African slaves of the island, it was incorporated into the voodoo belief system. The *loas* in modern practice include biblical figures as well as ancestral spirits. The most important aspect of voodoo is curing sick people.

Elephants in the Room

In Haitian culture, both in Haiti and particularly in the United States, it may be considered taboo to discuss voodoo practices. It may be the "elephant in the room" in clinical encounters with some Haitian American elders. Clinicians are advised to use sensitivity and open-ended questions when it is desirable or necessary to explore the use of voodoo practices with older Haitian American patients, because some of the deeply religious elders may be insulted by direct inquiry.

Mental illness may not be well-accepted by those adhering to traditional Haitian culture, and the use of mental health services may not be commonplace in some Haitian American families. Psychiatric illness is believed to be caused by supernatural factors such as hexes; as a result, a person suffering from depression or families of elder relatives with dementia may not come forward because of the social stigma. It is advisable to use sensitivity and diplomacy in exploring issues of mental health with older Haitian Americans and their families, and to incorporate traditional concepts of disease and wellness into treatment plans where indicated and appropriate.

Attitudes Toward North American Health Services

Traditional Haitian American elders may seek care from a North American health professional only when all other options involving traditional remedies or practitioners are exhausted. Infirmity is linked to not being able to work or be productive in the home, and the sick role is generally passive. Thus, North American clinicians may find that traditional Haitian American elders seek biomedical health care late in an illness. It is advisable to discuss each patient's attitudes and beliefs regarding professional visits early in the clinical relationship and to stress the importance of regular checkups for chronic health issues or prompt attention if new symptoms arise.

Traditionally, privacy and modesty are valued qualities in Haitian culture. Care should taken to ensure that procedures that require the older Haitian American to undress are adequately explained. Medical interpretation services should be incorporated into this process whenever necessary. If possible, in the interest of modesty, it is advisable to limit the removal of clothing only to the area that needs to be examined.

Traditionally, privacy and modesty are valued qualities in Haitian culture.

Culture-Specific Health Risks

Sexuality in the older Haitian is perceived to be outside culture and history. Interaction resulting in sexual relationships or diseases that are the product of sexual activity have nothing to do with society. Sexual relationships, if discussed at all, are talked about in the context of the marriage system. Haitian culture differs from Western culture in that approval of childhood sexual play, premarital sexuality, and same-sex coupling are not the norm in the Haitian community and are not addressed. These types of behaviors are considered shameful and inappropriate, such that they are simply ignored. Older Haitians tend to follow this standard. At least in this age group, sexuality should not be approached in the routine health encounter unless, of course, it is brought up by the patient. To approach the Haitian elder otherwise would demonstrate a lack of cultural sensitivity and could result in offending the patient quite deeply.

Behaviors associated with high risk in the United States may be viewed as unimportant by older Haitian Americans.

Behaviors associated with high risk in the United States may be viewed as unimportant by older Haitian Americans. For example, in Haitian culture, obesity is a sign of good health and being thin is associated with ill health. Older Haitian Americans may not emphasize the importance of exercise in the maintenance of good health and therefore may not exercise on a regular basis. Going to a gym is likely to be seen as a luxury, particularly by newer immigrants with limited financial means. In view of the reliance on self-care in traditional Haitian culture, the idea of seeing a physician for preventing health problems may not occur to the most recent older Haitian immigrants. As a result of some traditional attitudes toward health and well-being, some older recent Haitian immigrants may be at risk for undetected chronic health problems, such as hypertension, osteoarthritis, cerebrovascular disease, and cardiovascular disease.

Some older recent Haitian immigrants may be at risk for undetected chronic health problems.

Attempts to change the firmly held beliefs of an older Haitian American may be counterproductive to establishing a trusting doctor-patient relationship. Clinicians are advised to focus on establishing a strong, trusting, and flexible relationship with older Haitian patients and to negotiate slowly the needed changes to their health regime over the course of time.

Approach to Decision Making

Traditionally, the family system among Haitians is the core of life. The family includes not only members of the nuclear family but also relatives who are *consanguineous* (related by blood) and *affinal* (related by marriage). All may reside under the same roof. The family is involved with all aspects of a person's life, including education, marriage, calamity, and counseling. Each family has its own traditions, which form the basis for a family's reputation and are generalized to all members of the family. The reputation of a family is very significant and based on attributes such as honesty, pride, trust, social class, and history. For example, families who are experiencing financial difficulties may be well-respected if they are from a *grand famille* (important family). Families without a historical background are referred to as *nouveaux riches* (newcomers) and may find it difficult, even when they have money, to marry into a more well-established *grand famille*.

An important unit for decision making is the *conseil de famille* (family council). This council is generally composed of prominent members of the family, including the grandparents. The family structure is authoritarian and includes linear roles and responsibilities. Any action taken by one part of family has ramifications for the entire family. Esteem and shame are shared by all.

An important unit for decision making is the conseil de famille *(family council).*

It is common for Haitian Americans to have two equally involved family units: one in Haiti and one in the United States. Because of the paramount role the family plays in Haitian American life, it is advisable for clinicians early in the clinical relationship with a Haitian elder to establish the elder's preference regarding who should make his or her health decisions and under what circumstances. Clinicians may find Haitian families arriving at collective health decisions for an older family member, rather than having the capable elder make independent health decisions. When this is the case, it is useful to appoint a single family spokesperson to ensure ease of contact and continuity in communication.

Disclosure and Consent

The physician practicing in Haiti is considered to be an authority figure and is trusted to do what needs to be done without much consultation. As a result, clinicians in North America will find that Haitian American elders may not be familiar with current notions of informed consent in health decision making. Clinicians are advised to discuss this concept with older Haitian patients and, if requested, their family members, before embarking on the process of obtaining informed consent for clinical procedures.

Gender Issues

In traditional Haitian culture, gender responsibilities are well-defined and rigorously followed. Women are traditionally expected to fulfill subservient or supportive functions at home and in the workplace. Immigration to the United States may place strain on gender roles when both spouses must work to support a family and female family members are able to find employment more readily than their male partners. Such situations can result in reversal of traditional family roles, causing conflict in the extended family and difficulty in caring for older family members living at home and relying on female relatives for care. In traditional Haitian American families, supportive functions at home include nutrition, education, and health care, such that young women make decisions in these areas for themselves and their children.

> *In traditional Haitian culture, gender responsibilities are well-defined and rigorously followed.*

End-of-Life Decision Making and Care Intensity

When death is impending, it is common for an extended Haitian American family to gather for prayer and tears; commonly, religious medallions or other spiritual artifacts are incorporated into this ritual. When a person dies, an entire extended family is affected.

According to tradition, the oldest family member makes funeral arrangements and notifies the rest of the family. The body is not buried until the entire family can gather. The last bath is customarily given by a family member. In traditional Haitian culture, cremation is not considered, because interring the body is thought to be necessary for resurrection.

When death is impending, it is common for an extended Haitian American family to gather for prayer and tears.

Haitian Americans may prefer to die at home rather than in a hospital if at all possible. Autopsy is not prohibited, and if death is thought to be the result of malfeasance, an autopsy may be requested. An autopsy may also be requested to ensure that the body is actually dead and not a zombie. The word *zombie* refers to the voodoo belief that a *houngan* (voodoo priest) or *mambo* (voodoo priestess) can revive individuals who have died by causing a supernatural power to enter a dead body. After revival, the zombie is believed to remain under the control of the person who performed the ritual. Belief in zombies is more prevalent among older Haitian immigrants with rural backgrounds than among those who originated from larger cities. Because traditional Haitian Americans hold strong religious views about life after death, it is common for families to request that the body of a loved one remain intact for entombment. Family members of older Haitian Americans, therefore, may not be in favor of organ donation.

Use of Advance Directives

Most citizens of Haiti do not have access to hospitals offering resuscitation and ventilation, and the notion of do-not-resuscitate orders may not be familiar to some older Haitian immigrants who are less acculturated to the United States or who are newly arrived in the country.

However, clinicians working with large numbers of older Haitian Americans report that many of these patients are quite comfortable discussing end-of-life care and that those who are very religious may express the sentiment that the course at the end of life "is in God's hands." Clinicians working with older Haitian Americans are advised to raise the subject of preferences for care intensity in clinical discussions once trust has been built

between patient and provider and before critical medical problems arise. Descriptions from involved clinicians indicate that
when the patient-provider relationship is a trusting one, older
Haitians may request that decisions regarding care intensity be
left to the physician or clinician most involved with the patient.

Monica Stallworth, MD, MPH

| CASE STUDY **1** | **It's a Girl** |

Objectives
1. Develop culturally sensitive strategies to ensure effective cross-cultural interpersonal communication between provider and patient.
2. Respond to a Haitian American's cultural beliefs regarding food and disease.
3. Discuss strategies that include the family of a Haitian American patient and that respect their unique traits.

Dr. Worth is a middle-aged African American female geriatrician practicing in a world-renowned academic medical center. She is a sixth-generation American with a middle-class upbringing. She speaks no French or Haitian Creole.

Mr. Gabrey is a 71-year-old Haitian who has relocated to the United States to be with his daughter after the recent death of his wife. Mr. Gabrey was born in rural Haiti and comes from a background where resources were limited. He has managed to sustain himself in the United States with menial jobs. He lives with his daughter in a community of Haitian immigrants and is newly diagnosed with metastatic prostate cancer. Mr. Gabrey has been assigned to Dr. Worth.

Mr. Gabrey's primary language is Haitian Creole. He speaks limited English, and for this first encounter, his interpretation is through his daughter, Ariel, with whom he has lived since his wife's death.

His daughter has arranged the visit, because she has noticed that her father is not remembering well and she has found him talking to his deceased wife, especially before he goes to sleep.

Dr. Worth introduces herself to Mr. Gabrey while she is wearing regular "street" clothes and not carrying a stethoscope. Dr. Worth seats herself about 3 feet away facing Mr. Gabrey. She suggests that this first session should focus on her getting to know Mr. Gabrey. His daughter is agreeable. Although Dr. Worth addresses her questions to the patient, the daughter responds without consulting Mr. Gabrey, who sits quietly and looks down at the floor. Dr. Worth determines that it is best for the patient that she schedule a follow-up visit and use an interpreter upon his return.

Question:
1. What are the cultural issues that prevented communication in this encounter?

Mr. Gabrey returns for the follow-up visit; this time Dr. Worth is wearing her white coat and has her stethoscope. She has the interpreter, a male dressed in a white coat, sit next to Mr. Gabrey, who appears to be more comfortable. Dr. Worth uses open-ended questions about Mr. Gabrey's expectations of this encounter and how it differs from his experience in Haiti. She sits across from Mr. Gabrey and lets him direct the conversation. She also inquires about his wife's death and how his life has changed since that time. He mentions his problem with diarrhea since his wife's death and that he has trouble sleeping. He had tried to manage the diarrhea with "cold" food, but he can only tolerate small amounts of *akasan*. Dr. Worth asks permission to examine his abdomen. He agrees and he asks her to also listen to his heart.

Questions:
1. How would you respond to Mr. Gabrey's approach to managing his gastrointestinal symptoms with "cold" food and *akasan*?
2. What inference can you make about Mr. Gabrey's values, judging from the differences between his two clinical encounters with Dr. Worth?
2. How should Dr. Worth enlist the family to meet Mr. Gabrey's needs, physically and mentally?

This case study demonstrates the importance of the clinician's ability to assess the degree of acculturation of Haitian American elders, particularly with respect to their health care beliefs and expectations of health care professionals in clinical encounters. Each patient must be assessed individually, and effective clinicians will learn from their patients. Dr. Worth's sensitivity to Mr. Gabrey's beliefs will be all the more important when it comes to helping him and his family in making decisions about his end-of-life care and providing appropriate care for his cancer.

CASE STUDY **2**	**Sometimes I'm Listening but I Can't Hear You**

Objective

1. Discuss how the traditional Haitian concept of the real world—the natural and the supernatural—may impact end-of-life care for Haitian elders.

Dr. Steven is a geriatrician who is in private practice in Cambridge, Massachusetts, after taking over his father's practice 10 years ago. His family has been a part of the New England medical community for over 200 years. He continues to do inpatient medicine but is also dedicating a large portion of his time to hospital administration.

Mrs. Michele is 90 years old and Haitian born; she was brought in by her family to the emergency department after a fall. Unable to leave work for more than an hour, they leave Mrs. Michele alone in the emergency department. Mrs. Michele is admitted to Dr. Steven's service for work-up.

Mrs. Michele resides with three of her five children and their families. She also has a daughter who has returned to Haiti. Her son, deceased, was shot by a police officer in New York. Mrs. Michele was born in rural Haiti and has been in the United States for over 50 years. She did not complete grade school. She is functionally illiterate and communicates in Creole. She understands English and is able to say a few words, but until now she has lived in ethnic conclaves where Haitian Creole was the language spoken. Before her move to Cambridge, she worked as a housekeeper in Florida.

Dr. Steven does a standard work-up; imaging of Mrs. Michele's chest reveals probable lymphoma. He begins to discuss his suspicions with her, but she directs him to tell her family because she does not want to hear it. He informs her oldest daughter about the findings. When she attempts to tell her mother about the pulmonary mass, Mrs. Michele puts her hands over her ears.

Questions:

1. Why do you think that Mrs. Michele is resistant to any intervention or discussion of her disease?
2. Develop effective strategies that Dr. Steven might use to open the interpersonal communication between himself and Mrs. Michele so that a conversation can take place regarding her medical condition.

3. Discuss the level of acculturation of Mrs. Michele and how that might affect her ability to cope with her current crisis.

Dr. Steven contacts case management staff to arrange a family meeting to include all interested parties, including the patient. The patient agrees to participate on condition that her disease process is not directly discussed.

Mrs. Michele is the matriarch of her family; case management is concerned because they have 75 individuals confirmed to attend the family meeting, and all wish to have input. Dr. Steven enlists a Haitian American colleague, Dr. Simone Baptiste. They meet with Mrs. Michele to address underlying concerns. They do not discuss the disease by name, but she appears to be comfortable talking about her "illness" and "treatment." They find that Mrs. Michele believes that she needs to return to Haiti to address spiritual needs that orthodox medicine is not able to address here. She believes that her illness is simply the result of "imbalances" in her life at this time. Dr. Steven tells her that alternative therapies can be helpful but that he is not an expert in this area. Dr. Simone Baptiste concurs and says that she understands Mrs. Michele's desire to try ethnic medicine first.

Dr. Steven asks Mrs. Michele if she would be willing to have a conversation with the oncologist about possible treatment in Cambridge and dealing with its side effects. He suggests that perhaps there could be a combination of treatment that would satisfy her need to use the Haitian traditional treatment as well as the need for orthodox management. She says that she would like to have the family council involved in this decision. She agrees to talk with her family to reschedule the family meeting but limiting the number to six members of their own choosing.

Questions:
1. Develop strategies that the physicians might use in their meeting with Mrs. Michele and her family representatives.
2. Discuss the ways in which Mrs. Michele's concept of family might differ from that of her clinicians and how this difference might affect her health care.

To have genuine respect for a patient of a different culture and health beliefs, the culturally competent clinician must traverse values alien to his or her own, embracing different social systems and alternative decision-making styles. For older Haitians, cultural rituals and religious practices hold a great significance at times of illness. The sensitive clinician will facilitate the performance of important rituals whenever and to the extent possible to avoid creating or adding to unnecessary anxiety. In allowing Mrs. Michele and her family to choose six representatives to meet with her and the physicians treating her, Dr. Steven validated the involvement of the family, allowed for the possible use of alternative treatments along-side Western biomedical therapy, and even prepared the means for the possible appointment in the future of a health care proxy for Mrs. Michele.

References

Ackerman LK. Health problems of refugees. *J Am Board Fam Pract* 1997; 10(5):337–348.

Berggren WL, Ewbank DC, Berggren GG. Reduction of mortality in rural Haiti through a primary-health-care program. *New Eng J Med* 1981;304(22): 1324–1330.

Colin JM, Paperwalla G. Haitian-Americans. Available at: www-unix.oit.umass. edu/~efhayes/haitian.htm (accessed September 2005).

Colin JM, Paperwalla G. Haitians. In: Lipson JG, Dibble SL, Minarik PA, eds. *Culture and Clinical Care*. San Francisco: UCSF Nursing Press; 1996:139–154.

Corbett B. Introduction to Voodoo in Haiti. March 1988. Available at: www. webster.edu/~corbetre/haiti/voodoo/overview.htm (accessed September 2005).

Cruz GD, Shore R, Le Geros RZ, et al. Effect of acculturation on objective measures of oral health in Haitian immigrants in New York City. *J Dent Res* 2004;83(2):180–184.

De Santis L. Haitian immigrant concepts of health. *Health Values* 1993;17(6): 3–16.

De Santis L, Ugarriza DN. Potential for intergenerational conflict in Cuban and Haitian immigrant families. *Arch Psychiatric Nurs* 1995;9(6):354–364.

Gordon AM Jr. Caribbean basin refugees: the impact of Cubans and Haitians on health in South Florida. *J Fla Med Assoc* 1982;69(7):523–527.

Gustafson MB. Western voodoo: providing mental health care to Haitian refuges. *J Psychosoc Ment Health Serv* 1989;27(12):22–25.

Kemp C. Haitians. Available at: www3.baylor.edu/~Charles_Kemp/haitian_ refugees.htm (accessed September 2005).

Kiely SC, Grzybicki DM, Sepulveda A, et al. Chronic abdominal complaints and Helicobacter pylori in a Haitian population. *J Health Care Poor Underserved* 2004;15(2):183–192.

Laguerre MS. *American Odyssey: Haitians in New York City*. Ithaca, NY: Cornell University Press; 1984.

Laguerre MS. *Diasporic Citizenship: Haitian Americans in Transnational America*. New York: St. Martin's Press; 1998.

Miller NL. Haitian ethnomedical systems and biomedical practitioners: directions for clinicians. *J Transcult Nurs* 2000;11(3):204–211.

Molokhia M, Oakeshott P. A pilot study of cardiovascular risk assessment in Afro-Caribbean patients attending an inner city general practice. *J Fam Pract* 2000;17(1):60–62.

National Mental Health and Education Center. Understanding cultural issues in death. March 2003. Available at: www.naspcenter.org/principals/culture_ death.html (accessed September 2005).

Pierce WJ, Elisme E. Understanding and working with Haitian immigrant families. *J Fam Social Work* 1997;2(1):49–66.

Purnell LD, Paulanka BJ. Purnell's model for cultural competence. In: Purnell LD, Paulanka BJ, eds. *Transcultural Health Care: A Culturally Competent Approach*. Philadelphia: F.A. Davis Company; 1998:7–51.

Snow LF. Folk medical beliefs and their implications for care of patients: a review based on studies among black Americans. *Ann Intern Med* 1974;81(1):82–96.

Stepick A. *Pride Against Prejudice: Haitians in the United States*. Boston, MA: Allyn and Bacon; 1998.

U.S. Department of Health and Human Services. *Healthy People 2010: Understanding and Improving Health*. 2nd ed. Washington, DC: U.S. Government Printing Office; 2000.

Wilk RJ. The Haitian refugee: concerns for health care providers. *Soc Work Health Care* 1985–1986;11(2):61–74.

Zamor RC. *The Use of Herbal Remedies in Two Haitian Communities and Implications for Health-Care Providers Worldwide*. Lewiston, NY: Edwin Mellen Press; 2001.

Zéphir F. *Haitian Immigrants in Black America: A Sociological and Sociolinguistic Portrait*. Westport, CT: Bergin & Garvey; 1996.

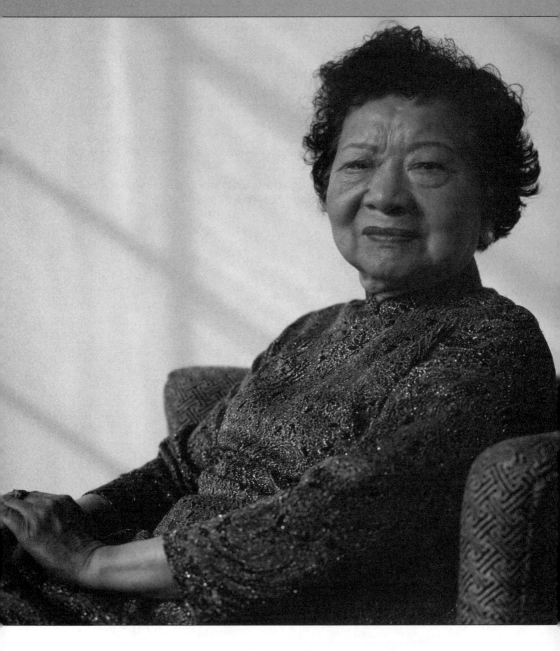

CHAPTER 6

Older Korean Americans

Doorway Thoughts

The influence of Confucianism in the Korean culture has resulted in a deep respect for education, authority, and filial piety. Confucianism is embedded in Korea's language and customs, and it is closely related to Koreans' traditional values and culture.

Older Korean Americans have a great sense of national pride in the United States, and at the same time they may have a strong sense of Korean ethnicity, in part because of the historical division of Korea into the North and the South.

Preferred Cultural Terms

The preferred term for the patient's cultural or ethnic identity is *Korean* or *Korean American.*

Formality of Address

Conversations with Korean American elders are customarily rather formal, reflecting the decorum and respect that is necessary in traditional Korean dialogue. Respect, especially respect for elders, is an important concept to be expressed during conversation. In traditional Korean culture, it is considered impolite to address a Korean elder by his or her first name. The appropriate form of address is Mr., Mrs., or Miss, followed by the individual's last name. In addition, Koreans traditionally accord respect to professionals such as physicians, and they may address physicians as *ui-sa*, a respectful term for "physician" or "doctor."

Respect, especially respect for elders, is an important concept to be expressed during conversation.

Language and Literacy

In Korea, most elders do not speak English, and Korean American elders in North America may not speak English even if they immigrated many years ago. This may be explained by a tendency to live in households with limited English proficiency, or possibly by living in communities where Korean language and culture predominate. One study in Los Angeles County revealed that 20 percent of the Korean American elders living there never spoke English; of those who did, 44 percent felt that they spoke it poorly. Although literacy rates among Korean American elders have not been explored fully, it is known that some elders are not literate in either Korean or English. Complicating the matter is the probability that some Korean elders, especially those with limited education, will not be forthright about their educational status or may even hide their illiteracy, because this may be a source of great embarrassment since education is very highly regarded in Korean culture.

Respectful Nonverbal Communication

During the medical interview with a Korean elder, it is advisable to convey an air of formality and respectfulness. Because of the influence of Confucianism in Korean culture, it is also important to show respect for the other person's sense of space during the conversation or examination.

Korean etiquette is complicated. It is considered polite to sit up straight in meetings and, when standing, to avoid putting one's hands into one's pockets. In conversation, extended direct eye contact may be considered impolite. Older Korean Americans who are less acculturated may not be accustomed to shaking hands, and it is advisable to maintain a conservative body language when first getting to know an elderly Korean patient. If one does shake hands, it is considered good manners to bow slightly at the same time.

> *If one does shake hands, it is considered good manners to bow slightly at the same time.*

History of Immigration

On January 13, 1903, the first group of Korean immigrants (56 men, 21 women, and 25 children) came to the island of Hawaii to work as laborers on sugar plantations. Before the 1960s, most Korean immigrants were uneducated laborers; after 1970 most were highly educated professionals or political refugees. Though initially Koreans resided in large metropolitan areas in the United States, presently newly immigrated Koreans are found in the suburbs and in the Southeast. Many of the recent older Korean immigrants to the United States have immigrated to join their adult children who immigrated earlier.

Degree of Acculturation

Because the history of Korean immigration to the United States spans more than a century, the degree of acculturation within the Korean American community varies widely. As with all older patients, it is important to ascertain each individual's cultural identification and preferences. Some Korean American elders have limited or no skills in English and may maintain traditional Korean customs, practices, social ties, and eating preferences. This will be more common among those elders who have immigrated recently to join children already living in North America. Other more recent immigrants may also be isolated from mainstream American culture, especially if they remain at home to take care of a household and grandchildren.

Some Korean American elders have limited or no skills in English and may maintain traditional Korean customs, practices, social ties, and eating preferences.

Tradition and Health Beliefs

Many Koreans, especially elders, prefer *Han bang*, also known as *Han yak*, a traditional form of Asian medicine, for their health care. Practitioners of traditional Asian medicine are called *Hanui*. *Han bang*, derived from Chinese traditional medical practices, is based on balance between *um* (the same as *yin*) and *yang*, as well as the balance of fire, earth, metal, water, and wood. Some diagnostic methods used in *Han bang* include observing the patient, obtaining a history of the illness, listening to a patient's voice, and taking the patient's pulse. The four most common treatment methods are acupuncture, herbs, moxibustion (direct or indirect burning with a stick made of the mugwort plant), and cupping (applying heated glass cups directly to the skin, forming a vacuum).

Older Koreans may attribute illnesses to a failure to fulfill spiritual obligations, whether these are based in Christianity, Confucianism, animism, or shamanism. Some may feel that their illnesses are due to failure to pray, others may attribute their illnesses to displeasure of ancestors with their burial place, or to having offended folk spirits. In one study of older Korean American women, the women attributed illnesses to *Hwabyung* ("fire illness"), caused by failing to keep their emotions from being expressed openly as traditionally required. Each emotion was believed to affect a particular organ system and the flow of *Ki* (the energy that animates all living things) in different ways. All of the women in the study were familiar with *Hwabyung,* and 80 percent, including those who were well educated, had experienced it. In most cases, it was related to difficult interpersonal or family relationships.

Older Korean Americans may alternate between seeing practitioners of Western and traditional Korean medicine. However, Korean elders may not readily discuss their experiences in the use of traditional Asian medicine with physicians trained in Western medicine, possibly because of a fear of ridicule or wish to avoid causing offense to the clinician. The astute clinician will inquire, in a supportive and respectful fashion, about beliefs concerning concepts of wellness and illness, as well as the use of traditional remedies. To be effective, treatment plans will most likely need to be negotiated, and they may need to include a mixture of Western and traditional practices.

Home Care and Food

In some Korean American families, parents will continue to live with the eldest son and rely on the son and daughter-in-law for financial and emotional support. Nursing homes exist in Korea but are rare, and in the United States, Korean Americans may not readily utilize nursing-home care. In households where both spouses are working, taking care of a frail elder at home may be a source of caregiver stress (often for the daughter-in-law). When elders' care needs exceed what can be realistically provided at home, this may also be a source of family and marital discord. In addition, if facility care is required, children may feel guilty that responsibilities toward a parent have not been fulfilled.

With regard to diet, rice is the main staple and is eaten with an array of side dishes featuring vegetables, fish, and meats. Fermented foods with soy sauce, bean paste, and red pepper were important sources of protein in early times and remain Korean favorites. In traditional Korean meals, numerous small servings of preserved foods are served. These foods are usually pickled in brine or packed in salt and lightly rinsed. Some Korean American elders are accustomed to eating Korean food for breakfast, lunch, and dinner. Some, however, often will have an American breakfast, consisting, for example, of fruit or cereal. In a survey of 208 older Korean Americans in Los Angeles County, 7.2 percent reported that their dietary pattern had changed a lot, 26.4 percent that it had changed somewhat, and 66.5 percent that their pattern had not really changed since living in the United States. About one half ate a Korean meal for breakfast, and almost 90 percent ate a Korean meal for dinner.

The traditional Korean diet is very high in salt. This high-salt diet predisposes individuals to hypertension and can be especially troublesome when patients with heart failure are noncompliant with their dietary restrictions. Dietary modification for health purposes will most likely require negotiation and gradual changes. Involvement of family members may be helpful, particularly those who do the cooking.

The traditional Korean diet is very high in salt.

Ethnic-Specific Health Risks

We have no national data on the health status and health service use of Korean elders. According to data from the Korea National Statistics Office, the major health problems of Korean elders in Korea include hypertension, cerebrovascular accidents, cancers (such as stomach or liver), and osteoporosis. Prevalence rates of infection with tuberculosis and hepatitis are higher in Korean Americans than in their European-descended counterparts. One study found that the infection rate among Korean adults with hepatitis B was 7 percent to 8 percent, compared with only 0.5 percent among white Americans. Rates of liver cirrhosis are consequently also higher. The rate of active tuberculosis infection in Korean American older persons is 12 times greater than it is among white Americans. There is also an increased risk for diabetes mellitus among older Korean Americans in comparison with the general U.S. population.

Health risks for Korean elders are further exacerbated by the fact that large numbers of Koreans lack health insurance. One out of every three Korean Americans in the United States is uninsured, whereas 21 percent of all Asian American and Pacific Islanders and 14 percent of non-Latino whites are uninsured. In Los Angeles County, where a large number of Koreans reside, the proportion of the uninsured is more than 40 percent. Korean American older persons may be less aware of available long-term health and social services than members of other minority ethnic groups in the United States.

> *Korean American older persons may be less aware of available long-term health and social services than members of other minority ethnic groups in the United States.*

A larger proportion of older Korean Americans consider themselves to be in poor health when compared with the general population. Without health insurance, preventive health care is substantially more challenging to access for elders in this population. Improving access to health services may be impeded by a relative lack of research with older Korean Americans, in comparison with research in other minority populations of similar size.

Approaches to Decision Making

Ideas of individualism and autonomy are unfamiliar in traditional Korean culture. Korean culture emphasizes the individual as a part of a family unit, and decisions are made collectively by family groups. Korean elders will often involve family members in decision making, and an important health decision will commonly involve their conferring with and relying on an eldest son, if one exists. Attitudes toward decision making in a context of serious illness are discussed in the next section.

Attitudes Regarding Disclosure and Consent

According to several published studies, traditional Korean Americans may not be in favor of direct disclosure or consent at times of serious illness. Some Korean Americans believe that voicing thoughts about sickness or death will contribute to a poor outcome when someone has a life-threatening illness. Similarly, some Koreans believe that once a terminal diagnosis has been disclosed, the person who is sick may become depressed and lose the will to live. Older Korean Americans may believe that only the family, and not the patient, should be told about a terminal diagnosis. In this family-centered model, it is the responsibility of the family to hear bad news about the patient's diagnosis and prognosis, and to make the difficult decisions about investigations, treatment, and end-of-life care. As a result, when Korean Americans have a grave illness, they may not favor being told directly of the terminal diagnosis or prognosis, and they may prefer to assign responsibility for their own health decision making to family members. The skillful clinician will discuss preferences regarding truth telling, disclosure, consent, and decision making with an older patient early in the clinical relationship, and then confirm these wishes at intervals.

Older Korean Americans may believe that only the family, and not the patient, should be told about a terminal diagnosis.

When families are called upon to make health decisions for an elder, there may be conflict between family members with differing views. In such instances, either asking the patient to assign a principal decision maker or asking the family in a group meeting to assign a primary spokesperson will enhance communication and assist in reaching optimal health decisions for the patient.

Gender Issues

Traditional Korean society is patriarchal, and until recently, it was common for Korean women to stay at home to take care of the family. Korean immigrant families commonly have had to change abruptly from having a single income provider to situations where the women are also working outside of the home. This may be a source of conflict for a Korean American family if the husband resents it when his wife is also a family breadwinner. Korean women may feel burdened if they have to continue to perform all the household-related work in addition to their responsibilities in the workplace.

Even highly acculturated Korean Americans may regard it as natural for adult children to be responsible for aging parents and to provide care for them at home. Women customarily are the caregivers to home-dwelling Korean American elders. Provision of such care at home can be both emotionally and financially draining; even the closest and most supportive families are at risk for caregiver stress and burnout. Although present in all cultures, such situations in the Korean American community may result in high degrees of burden when caregivers feel the traditional pressures of providing all elder care personally and within the home setting. Clinicians working with Korean Americans are advised to be sensitive to the potential for caregiver distress and to provide support to elders and caregivers well in advance of a crisis situation for the patient and family.

End-of-Life Decision Making and Care Intensity

Decisions regarding end-of-life issues and intensity of medical care are often influenced by religious beliefs, personal beliefs, and also beliefs related to ethnicity and culture. In the traditional Korean family, the eldest son usually will be expected to make decisions regarding his parents' end-of-life care. As discussed in the section on disclosure and consent, Korean American elders may prefer not to make their own health decisions when life-threatening illness is diagnosed.

Attitudes Toward Advance Directives

Decisions and discussions regarding advance directives may be difficult because they also involve raising issues of death and dying. Koreans, like those from other ethnic groups, commonly believe that discussing death directly when a person is terminally ill will bring about sadness or depression and hasten death. Nevertheless, discussions of advance directives are important, even if a patient (or the designated family decision maker) prefers not to express his or her wishes in writing. In one study looking at the relationship between ethnicity and advance directives in a frail older population, Asians were found to be more likely than whites

> *In the traditional Korean family, the eldest son usually will be expected to make decisions regarding his parents' end-of-life care.*

to select less aggressive interventions but were unlikely to use written directives. As discussed in the section on disclosure and consent, older Korean Americans may assign family members as their primary health decision makers; such individuals should be involved as much as possible in defining an appropriate approach to care for each older Korean patient.

Linda Sohn, MD, MPH

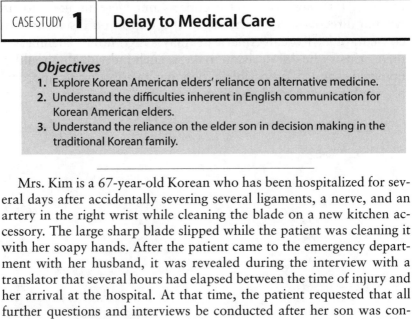

CASE STUDY **1** | **Delay to Medical Care**

Objectives

1. Explore Korean American elders' reliance on alternative medicine.
2. Understand the difficulties inherent in English communication for Korean American elders.
3. Understand the reliance on the elder son in decision making in the traditional Korean family.

Mrs. Kim is a 67-year-old Korean who has been hospitalized for several days after accidentally severing several ligaments, a nerve, and an artery in the right wrist while cleaning the blade on a new kitchen accessory. The large sharp blade slipped while the patient was cleaning it with her soapy hands. After the patient came to the emergency department with her husband, it was revealed during the interview with a translator that several hours had elapsed between the time of injury and her arrival at the hospital. At that time, the patient requested that all further questions and interviews be conducted after her son was contacted, since neither the patient nor her husband spoke English. When consenting to medical care, the patient also requested that all decisions regarding her care be made by her son.

The patient was admitted to the hospital, and surgery was performed emergently to stop the bleeding and repair the nerves and ligaments, in an attempt to preserve functioning. At the time of the surgery, the patient and her family were told that the function of the right hand might not be fully restored because many hours had elapsed before she had sought medical care.

Question:

1. What culturally related issues may have prevented the patient from receiving timely medical care?

Later, upon further questioning, it is revealed that precious time had elapsed while the patient and her husband drove around Korea town in Los Angeles seeking medical attention from two other providers before coming to the hospital emergency department. They first went to see a practitioner who specializes in herbal medicine. After learning that she could not be treated there, the patient and her husband went to another physician, who directed them to the emergency department. The patient states that prior to immigrating to the United States over 20 years ago and currently, her usual source of medical care has been from practitioners of complementary and alternative medicine (CAM). Not only is she more comfortable with the use of CAM, she finds that talking with a health provider who speaks Korean to be much easier. She admits that she is embarrassed by the fact that she and her husband cannot speak English and that they use CAM; she also says that they are worried about the cost of medical care in the hospital since they do not have health insurance.

Question:

1. How will discussions about the use of CAM improve communication with the patient and better prepare the patient for discharge and rehabilitation?

After the surgery and several days of recuperation, plans are made for discharge from the hospital. The physician in charge tells the patient and her son that in addition to many months of rehabilitation to regain functioning of the right wrist that they will need to follow up with a physician. They are told that it will be important to follow the progress of improvement with rehabilitation but also to coordinate her rehabilitation with appropriate care with CAM, if they so desire.

| CASE STUDY **2** | **Conflict Between East and West** |

Objectives
1. Discuss the conflicts between complementary and alternative medicine (CAM) and Western medicine.
2. Understand the implications of the lack of health insurance for both the patient and the clinician.
3. Discuss the impact on patients' health of the lack of preventive medical care.

Mrs. Han is a 72-year-old Korean who is brought to the emergency department for altered mental status. The patient has come to the nearest county hospital because she does not have health insurance. Initially, laboratory tests reveal an elevated corrected hypercalcemia of 16.0, elevated BUN of 50, and elevated serum creatinine of 2.3. On physical examination, it is revealed that the patient had a 2.0-cm mass in the right upper quadrant of the left breast. The patient's altered mental status improves after correction of her electrolyte abnormalities with intravenous fluids. Because the patient does not speak English, a translator is used to gather a more in-depth medical history. The patient immigrated to the United States 15 years ago and has lived with her eldest son since her husband passed away. Though she frequents alternative medicine clinics for medical care, she has never before sought Western medical care in the United States. She states that she has never had a mammogram or clinical breast examination. She does not know how to perform a self-examination of her breast.

Later the next day, her son arrives at the hospital. After learning about her condition and medical treatment, he becomes very agitated and asks to speak to the physicians in charge of her care. The son is adamantly opposed to the use of the intravenous fluids and wants to start cupping (a CAM treatment) for his mother during her hospitalization. The patient's son states that he is an alternative medicine practitioner. He believes that the intravenous fluids are drawing the life force out of his mother.

Question:
1. How could the conflict between alternative and Western medicine be handled appropriately?

The physician in charge of the case confers with the patient. After first determining that her sensorium has cleared and that she is able to make decisions for herself and her health care, he questions her. She states that she would like her son to make all decisions regarding her medical care. The son is informed that the medical team has concluded that the cause of her altered mental status is the electrolyte imbalance in her body, which was caused by the palpable mass in the patient's left breast, mostly likely breast cancer. However, further blood tests, radiologic studies, and soft-tissue biopsy will be needed to confirm the diagnosis. The patient's son is greatly concerned about the intravenous fluids and asks that they be discontinued; he also wishes to start the practice of cupping. When the patient's son is questioned regarding the cupping, he explains that it consists of using cups to apply suction to the skin to apply heat. The son and his mother are told that the practice cannot be performed in the hospital because of the potential fire hazard, especially since oxygen tanks are often present in the hospital ward. It is agreed that the intravenous fluids will be discontinued, but it is explained that this most certainly will result in the patient's losing consciousness again and perhaps dying. The son responds by declaring that he would like to have his mother discharged from the hospital so that he can begin the cupping therapy at home.

Question:

1. How could assistance be provided to this patient and family prior to discharge?

Prior to her discharge from the hospital, the patient and her son are referred to the social worker. The social worker gives them information about community health care clinics that serve the Korean American population. She also gives them a contact number for a community social worker from whom they will be able to obtain information about Medicaid and Medicare.

References

Andersen R, Harada N, Chiu V, et al. Application of the behavioral model to health studies of Asian and Pacific Islander Americans. *Asian Am Pac Isl J Health* 1995;3(2):128–141.

Blackhall LJ, Murphy ST, Frank G, et al. Ethnicity and attitudes toward patient autonomy. *JAMA* 1995;274(10):820–825.

Chow M. Korean American history. Available at: www.asianweek.com/2003_01_10/feature_timeline.html (accessed November 2005).

Commonwealth Fund. Minority Americans lag behind whites on nearly every measure of health care quality. Press release. March 2002. Available at: www.cmwf.org/newsroom/newsroom_show.htm?doc_id=223608 (accessed November 2005).

Eleazer GP, Hornung CA, Egbert CB, et al. The relationship between ethnicity and advance directives in a frail older population. *J Am Geriatr Soc* 1996;44(8):938–943.

Kagawa-Singer M, Hikoyeda N, Tanjasiri SP. Aging, chronic conditions, and physical disabilities in Asian and Pacific Islander Americans. In: Markides KS, Miranda MR, eds. *Minorities, Aging and Health*. Thousand Oaks, CA: Sage Publications; 1997:149–175.

Kim M, Han HR, Kim KB, et al. The use of traditional and Western medicine among Korean American elderly. *J Community Health* 2002;27(2):109–120.

Moon A, Lubben JE, Villa V. Awareness and utilization of community long-term care services by elders Korean and non-Hispanic white Americans. *Gerontologist* 1998;38(3):309–316; discussion 317–319.

Pang KY. The practice of traditional Korean medicine in Washington D.C. *Soc Sci Med* 1989;28:875–884.

Shin KR, Shin C, Blanchette PL. Health and health care of Korean-American elders. Available at: www.stanford.edu/group/ethnoger/index.html (accessed November 2005).

Sohn L. The health and health status of older Korean Americans at the 100-year anniversary of Korean immigration. *J Cross Cult Gerontol* 2004;19(3):203–219.

Tanjasiri SP, Wallace SP, Shibata K. Picture imperfect: hidden problems among Asian Pacific islander elderly. *Gerontologist* 1995;35(6):753–760.

Yoon AS. Long term care for the Korean-American elderly. Available at: www.icasinc.org/2000/2000m/2000masy.html (accessed November 2005).

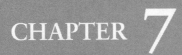

CHAPTER 7

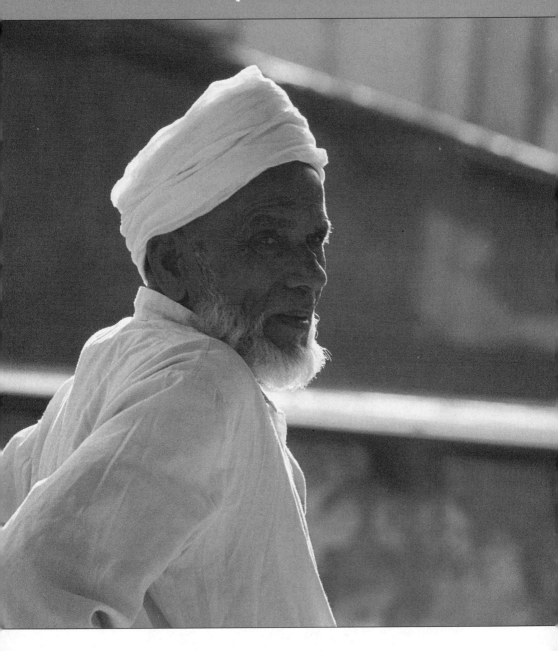

Older Pakistani Americans

Doorway Thoughts

Older Pakistani adults in the United States are diverse in both traditional values and religious beliefs. The four provinces of Pakistan have distinct cultural and language differences, and immigrants to North America are consequently a heterogeneous group in culture, language, and socioeconomic status. There are two distinct groups of Pakistani elders in the United States: The first consists of the parents or grandparents who immigrated with their children; this chapter primarily addresses the needs of this group. The second group consists of the professionals who immigrated to this country in the 1950s and 1960s; their acculturation is very different from that of the first group. Given the length of their acculturation, their communication skills and clinical adherence will differ from their parents' and grandparents'.

Although elders from Pakistan who have migrated to the United States may not all be Muslims, the majority of Pakistani American elders will identify Islam as their religion. For this reason, Islam is used as the religious norm for this chapter. However, as is recommended for all cultural groups discussed in the *Doorway Thoughts* series, the clinician should ask about each patient's religious preference and not assume that every Pakistani American elder is Muslim.

Preferred Cultural Terms

The preferred term for Americans with roots in Pakistan is *Pakistani American,* regardless of their province of origin in Pakistan.

Attitudes Toward North American Health Services

The following questions, when asked of a Pakistani American older patient, may guide the clinician in determining how the elder conceives of health, illness, and health care:

- What do you call the problem?

- Why do you think this illness or problem has occurred? (For example, the Pakistani American patient may feel that the problem is a punishment given by God for bad deeds committed or that it is due to a magic spell.)

- What do you think the illness does? (For example, the patient may feel that the illness is washing away her or his sins and will resolve once the sins are cleansed, or when certain religious rituals have been are performed.)

- What do you think is the natural course of the illness? What do you fear? (For example, patients may either have undue fear of the disease, or conversely, may trivialize the disease and feel that it can be resolved by prayer. It is important to understand the patient's bias so that appropriate education can be provided.)

- How do you think the sickness should be treated? What alternative therapies are you using currently? How do want us to help you? (These questions should be asked in a way that avoids creating the impression that the clinician lacks confidence or competence. Once a patient's expectations are known, a specific care plan can be devised.)

- Who do you turn to for help? Who should be involved in decision making? (Pakistani Americans may have a close-knit family structure, and the family unit often makes important decisions.)

Formality of Address

Old age is highly respected in Pakistan. In Pakistani culture, older people are treated with extreme respect and are never called by their first name, especially by younger persons. Patients should be addressed formally, using the correct title (e.g., Mr. or Mrs.). Older Pakistani patients may use the doctor's first name with title (e.g., Dr. Amna or Dr. David).

Language and Literacy

Pakistani American older adults may not speak English (especially the women) and may be able to converse only in Urdu or a dialect (e.g., Punjabi). Urdu (derived mainly from Arabic, Persian, and Hindi vocabulary) is the national language of Pakistan. If an Urdu interpreter is unavailable, an interpreter speaking Hindi may be helpful, because Urdu and Hindi are similar languages. Usually, younger relatives who can serve as interpreters accompany their elders. However, the use of family interpreters is controversial, because information may be changed or eliminated by family for a variety of reasons (disagreement, embarrassment, or level of acculturation). It is advisable to use professional interpreters periodically just to make sure that all of the patient's concerns are being addressed. This is especially true for elderly women who are brought by their male relatives and out of modesty may not talk about intimate personal details. Same-sex professional interpreters are preferred.

> *It is advisable to use professional interpreters periodically just to make sure that all of the patient's concerns are being addressed.*

Pakistani American patients will customarily hold the clinician in high regard, so much so that they may not divulge information that they consider to be unnecessary or burdensome in front of an interpreter or directly to the clinician. The culturally sensitive clinician will gently encourage and support these older patients and assure absolute confidentiality of the clinical interview and medical records.

Respectful Nonverbal Communication

Elderly Pakistani Americans may wear religious paraphernalia; examples include the *taawiz* (amulet) or *topi* (religious cap worn by men). These should not be removed without the permission of the owner.

Pakistani American older adults may be accompanied by a relative, who most likely will display an attitude of respect and deference toward the patient and will expect clinicians to do the same. Gestures of respect include opening doors and standing when the older patient enters the room.

Pakistani older adults are used to a very formal approach by their physicians and may be taken aback by a more informal approach, especially by physical contact other than that required for a clinical examination. Physical contact (touching and holding hands) in the clinical encounter is uncommon, even when initiated by a same-sex clinician. It is appropriate for a male clinician to shake hands with men. Physical contact between opposite sexes is prohibited in some Pakistani communities, and some female patients may not feel comfortable shaking hands with either male or

It is advised that clinicians adopt a formal body language in early encounters with Pakistani elders,

female clinicians. It is advised that clinicians adopt a formal body language in early encounters with Pakistani elders, and that they ascertain acceptable forms of physical contact early in the clinical relationship.

Physicians in particular are traditionally expected to be self-assured figures of authority. Informality may not be the best approach to developing a relationship with older Pakistani American patients. Clinicians are advised to start by adopting a demeanor that is warm and caring while at the same time formal and reserved, and to take cues from the patient regarding comportment and formality as the clinical relationship develops.

History of Immigration

Some immigrants from Pakistan may have arrived after the 1947 partition of the subcontinent, but a larger wave of immigrants came after 1965, the year President Lyndon Johnson sponsored an immigration bill that repealed the longstanding system of quotas by national origin. Under the new system, preferences went to relatives of U.S. residents and those with special occupational skills needed in the United States. Although Pakistanis have been a small part of the immigrant population of the United States all through the 20th century, in recent decades their ranks have grown significantly.

According to the 2000 U.S. Census, 16,978 individuals identified themselves as Pakistani Americans and as being 55 years old or older. About 96.7 percent identified themselves as having been born outside United States. In 1995 elderly Pakistani women (52.1%) slightly outnumbered the men (47.9%). Between 1989 and 1992, a total of 2433 elders over the age of 60 years emigrated from Pakistan to the United States.

Pakistanis, many of whom are skilled professionals such as doctors and engineers, have played an important role in the development of Muslim community groups in the United States and in lay leadership of mosque communities.

Degree of Acculturation

Most of the Pakistani older adults currently seeking care in the United States are recent immigrants who have moved here to be closer to their children. Such elders may be mostly dependent on their children for transportation and socialization, and they may socialize primarily with other South Asian immigrants. In addition, these patients may subscribe to a traditional health belief system and have little relation to Western mainstream health practices. This patient cohort will likely differ socially from the cohort of Pakistani Americans who are now older but who immigrated to the United States in the 1960s. Individuals in this latter group are likely to be more acculturated to North American cultural and health practices. The astute clinician will inquire, rather than assume, about each individual patient's cultural preferences and approaches.

> *These patients may subscribe to a traditional health belief system and have little relation to Western mainstream health practices.*

Traditional Health Beliefs

The majority of the Pakistani American elders are used to "mixing" the health care systems. They use Western medicine for some ailments while still holding on to their traditional belief system. Muslims also believe that the time of death is fixed by Allah and ultimate healing is in Allah's hands. Maintaining spiritual peace is thought to be an essential part of health. Elderly immigrants who are bound to traditions may believe that disease can be a direct punishment by God for sins committed. Following religious teachings and not doing evil, therefore, is viewed as an integral part of staying healthy. Elders, especially women, initially may try traditional folk medicine when illness strikes. They may then seek allopathic medical help only when the suffering due to the disease becomes intolerable or when they are forced to by younger family members.

> *Maintaining spiritual peace is thought to be an essential part of health.*

Health beliefs of older Pakistani American are a combination of Muslim faith and traditional cultural practices from the Indian subcontinent that have been passed on for thousands of years. *Hikmat* (literally meaning "wisdom") or *Unani* (literally meaning "Greek") medicine are the traditional health systems most commonly used in Pakistan. *Hikmat* is a form of therapy based on the Greek humoral theory of Hippocrates. The *Unani* system is based on the Hippocratic theory that a perfect balance of *arkan* (elements), *akhlat* (humors), and *mizaj* (temperament) helps in keeping the body and mind healthy. Every individual is believed to have an inherent power of self-preservation called the *Quwat-e-Modabira*. The theory assumes the presence of four humors in the human body: *dum* (blood), *balgham* (phlegm), *safra* (yellow bile), and *saoda* (black bile).

It is believed diseases are caused when the functions associated with the vital, natural, and psychic forces of the body become obstructed or unbalanced, owing to a deviation in a humor away from its characteristic temperament. The *hakim* (*Unani* practitioner), after identifying the imbalance, will often recommend, among other things, appropriate foods that are specifically chosen to correct the imbalance and restore equilibrium. *Hakims* are given great importance in the Pakistani health belief system, and even educated people sometimes prefer to go to a *hakim* for their health care.

> Homeopathic medicine is also well respected among Pakistani people.

Homeopathic medicine is also well respected among Pakistani people. Homoeopathy is based on the Law of Cure, namely, "like cures like." This field was started by a German physician, Dr. Samuel Hahnemann, in 1796. The remedies are prepared from natural substances and are thought to work by stimulating the body's own healing power.

When ill, religious Muslims may wear the *taawiz*, an amulet containing verses from the Koran. The *taawizes* are symbols of Islamic faith, given by the *pirs* (holy men) and worn by adults to cure and prevent illness caused by the evil eye, black magic, ghosts, or evil spirits.

Consultations with the *pir* and visits to shrines and tombs (*pir's ziarat gahh*) are believed to prevent and cure many physical and mental illnesses, including those caused by ghosts and spirits. Holy water from *pirs'* tombs can be imbibed or rubbed on the body of the sick. Some people also use butter or oil blessed by the *pir* and rub it on the area of pain or tumor. These practices vary by education, social class, and degree of religious fervor. Many individuals from professional families lean toward Western medical practices and do not visit shrines.

Hand washing is considered essential before and after eating. Water for washing is needed in the same room as the toilet; Pakistani patients should be provided with bowls or jugs of water in the bathroom. If a bedpan has to be used, bowls or jugs of water should also be provided at the bedside. Pakistani American Muslims may also pray five times a day, and they need to wash all exposed parts of their body before each prayer. Many older Pakistani American patients who are traditional Muslims will attend the *masjid* (mosque or Islamic place of worship) on Fridays to offer special prayers. The sensitive clinician will be aware of this religious responsibility and avoid, whenever possible, scheduling appointments or tests during Friday prayers.

> *Pakistani American Muslims may also pray five times a day, and they need to wash all exposed parts of their body before each prayer.*

Psychiatric diseases are considered taboo in many Pakistani communities. Individuals may feel embarrassed to seek treatment for depression or psychosis, for fear of being labeled *pagul* or crazy. Such subjects should be tackled with great tact, sensitivity, and discretion.

Home Care and Food

Religious Muslims eat only *halal* (lawful or sanctified meat) and do not eat blood products, pork, or *haram* (nonsanctified) meat. Most Pakistani American elders will follow these dietary laws. If halal meals are not available, kosher or vegetarian meals are acceptable. Alcohol is also prohibited in Islam, and most Pakistani Americans, especially older women, will not drink alcohol or eat food prepared with alcohol-based products.

> *If halal meals are not available, kosher or vegetarian meals are acceptable.*

Because many Pakistani Americans try to avoid all pork products, they may not want to take certain medications containing animal pectin or gelatin. Also, it is advisable to avoid using porcine insulin and other pork-based products for Pakistani patients.

Every year during the month of Ramadan (called *Ramzan* in Pakistan), Pakistani American Muslims fast from first daylight until sunset. Fasting is regarded spiritually as a method of self-purification. This obviously has implications for the frail elders and people with diabetes mellitus. Sick and elderly believers may be exempt from fasting during Ramzan; some exceptions are made for frail individuals. Clinicians are advised to discuss practices during Ramzan with their older Pakistani patients and to negotiate a safe care plan early in the clinical relationship.

Pakistani food varies from region to region, but most of it is curry-based and spicy. It is similar to North Indian food served in many Indian or Pakistani restaurants in North America. Dietary staples include meat- and vegetable-based curry and basmati rice or *chapatti* (unleavened whole wheat bread). Pakistani food has high salt and fat content. Most of Pakistani American older adults will find the U.S. hospital food bland and tasteless and may ask family members to bring food from home.

There are no nursing homes in Pakistan, and traditionally families want to provide care for their families at home. It may be considered shameful for a family to send their elder to a nursing home.

Culture-Specific Health Risks

Pakistani Americans overall are at high risk for coronary heart disease, hypertension, dyslipidemia, and diabetes mellitus. Other prevalent health problems include tuberculosis (for patients born in Pakistan), oral submucous fibrosis (often secondary to chewing *paan*, which is betel quid with added spices), and oral cancers (patients with submucous fibrosis who also smoke are at high risk). Pakistani immigrant women in the United States are at higher risk for breast cancer than their counterparts in Pakistan.

Pakistani Americans overall are at high risk for coronary heart disease, hypertension, dyslipidemia, and diabetes mellitus.

Although there are no data available for Pakistanis living in the United States, depression is found to be highly prevalent in Pakistan (44%) and among Pakistanis living in the United Kingdom (42%). Adverse social circumstances are believed to be the cause of these findings. High-risk health behaviors of Pakistani elders include high-fat diets, a high prevalence of smoking and chewing tobacco by the men, and a sedentary lifestyle.

Attitudes Regarding Disclosure and Consent

Some Pakistani American families may ask the clinician not to disclose a diagnosis to a patient, especially when it involves cancer. As discussed in the first chapter, bioethical guidelines allow for individual patients to assign their decision-making rights to another individual or group, and it is generally agreed that incorporating patients' wishes regarding disclosure and consent into clinical planning is beneficial. Some patients may prefer not to know if they are terminally ill and ask that family members or other caregivers receive all diagnostic information and make all treatment decisions. It is advisable to explore each patient's preferences regarding disclosure of serious clinical findings early in the clinical relationship and to reconfirm these wishes at intervals.

Saying something like, "Mr. Qureshi, I am told that you prefer to let your family make all health care decisions for you and that you would prefer not to know your diagnosis. Is this correct?" will help confirm the patient's stance.

Gender Issues

Female professionals are customarily the preferred service providers for elderly Pakistani women. Older women may prefer not to disrobe even for professionals of their own sex, and they may need a lot of gentle reassurance during the clinical examination.

Many older Pakistani American women may prefer to defer decision making to their husband, sons, or daughters. Older Pakistani men may be more independent in their decision making but still defer to their children for certain decisions.

Questions about sexuality are considered extremely delicate and personal issues. Therefore, questions about sexuality should be asked with particular sensitivity. Asking a widowed woman about her sex life is a cultural faux pas and can be taken as a significant insult. Older women may prefer not to change into a gown, even when the clinician is a woman. Clinicians

Asking a widowed woman about her sex life is a cultural faux pas and can be taken as a significant insult.

are advised to explain clearly and gently the necessity of using a gown and appropriate drapes to enhance the efficacy of the clinical examination, and to adopt a demeanor of formality and deferential support during all examinations and procedures.

Pakistani men have been used to being in a leadership role in society, and they may therefore have a difficult time coping with disability and dependence on others.

End-of-Life Decision Making and Advance Directives

Active end-of-life care planning is an unfamiliar concept to most Pakistani American families.

Active end-of-life care planning is an unfamiliar concept to most Pakistani American families. Clinicians who have discussions about advance directives and advance care planning should remember that the elders might be reluctant to participate in these discussions, because they may believe that talking about death will make it a reality. Worse, the elders may believe that the clinician is subtly implying that they have a serious illness and are dying. Particular tact and sensitivity are called for when having these conversations. It is advisable to ensure that the clinician has adequate time for end-of-life conversations, and that a patient's family is present. This is also an appropriate time to consider involving a professional medical interpreter in the clinical encounter.

In Islam, withholding food is forbidden. Providers should therefore be very sensitive to issues regarding withdrawal of tube feedings.

Pakistani older adults most commonly wish to die at home, surrounded by their family and community members. When this is requested, the sensitive clinician may wish to facilitate a patient's return home, to be cared for until death.

Whether at home or in a hospital, a Pakistani American patient may expect to have family and friends gathered around for a final farewell when death is approaching. This is traditionally an important event in the Pakistani community, allowing a dying person to put right, before death, anything he or she feels is wrong in relationships with family, friends, or community. Visiting the sick is a sacred duty according to Islam, as well as a last opportunity to show respect to a fellow Muslim and the family.

The hospitalized Pakistani patient may have more visitors than the health care team expects; for example, more than 20 visitors a day is not uncommon. Many of these visitors will also want to assist in the patient's care. Sensitivity on the part of staff may be required in coaching family and friends as to how they may, and may not, assist at the bedside. Family and friends may wish to read passages from the Koran to the patient, and prayers for forgiveness for any past sins may also be said.

Sensitivity on the part of staff may be required in coaching family and friends as to how they may, and may not, assist at the bedside.

Traditional Muslims have extensive death rituals, including ceremonial washing of the body with holy waters, directional positioning of the body toward the holy city of Mecca, and immediate burial procedures. If no family or friends are present when the patient dies, it is best to close the eyes, cover the body with a white sheet, and turn the body on its right side facing southeast. The health care worker should wash only body fluids or excrement from the body. There is a ritual washing of the body performed by Muslims of the same sex as the deceased as soon as possible. If possible, same-sex providers should handle the body and try to avoid physical contact as much as possible. As Muslims believe that there is still "awareness" after death, post-mortem examinations are disliked, and if recommended, may cause great anxiety for the family.

Traditional Muslims have extensive death rituals, including ceremonial washing of the body with holy waters, directional positioning of the body toward the holy city of Mecca, and immediate burial procedures.

Amna B. Buttar, MD, MS
Jennifer C. Mendez, PhD
Vyjeyanthi S. Periyakoil, MBBS, MD

| CASE STUDY **1** | **End-of-Life Decision Making** |

Objectives

1. Understand and explain possible bases of resistance by Pakistani family members to disclosure of diagnoses of terminal illness to older patients.
2. List potential strategies that could be used with Pakistani elders and family members in cases of lack of agreement on end-of-life care.

Mr. Chaudhry, a 70-year-old Pakistani, is brought to the outpatient clinic for evaluation of gait unsteadiness. He has been diagnosed with lung cancer with metastases to the liver. His wife passed away 6 months ago, and he moved to America because all his children have settled here. He is a farmer from Punjab and speaks only Punjabi. A left hemiparesis is found during the examination, and the internist wants to get a computed tomography (CT) scan of the head to exclude brain metastases. The patient's eldest son, Manzoor, who also serves as his interpreter, accompanies Mr. Chaudhry and says that he is the primary decision maker for his father. Mr. Chaudhry confirms this statement.

The son takes the doctor aside and requests that she should not tell the patient about her suspicion of brain metastases. The son agrees with getting the tomography and obtaining a radiation oncology and oncology consult but asks that all these doctors not mention "cancer" as they discuss treatment. He thinks that if his father learns about the possibility of cancer in the brain, he will give up the will to live. The son still believes that his father will be cured of the cancer. In addition to the allopathic treatment, the family is also consulting a spiritual healer in Pakistan, who has assured them that the cancer will be cured in 6 months.

The CT scan of the head shows a large brain mass on the right side that is causing cerebral edema and midline shift. Mr. Chaudhry is started on oral corticosteroids and radiation therapy. The spiritual healer has given the family oil that is blessed by holy words, and they apply it to his head, chest, back, and abdomen. Mr. Chaudhry develops dermatitis on the scalp and is told by the radiation oncologist not to use this "hair oil." The patient stops eating and drinking and becomes very weak; he is admitted to the hospital.

Question:

1. How could you address the lack of cultural competence of the radiation oncologist who tells the family not to use the oil blessed by holy words, calling it "hair oil"?

You are concerned that if the family feels insulted because of the oncologist's lack of understanding, it could affect the trust relationship you have built with Mr. Chaudhry and his family. After explaining to your colleague the importance of being sensitive to the religious beliefs for healing of families from diverse backgrounds, you organize a meeting of you and the oncologist with Mr. Chaudhry and family members. The two of you explore with family members their explanation of the use and meaning of the oil given to them by the spiritual healer. After hearing their description of the importance to them of the healing function of the oil, the radiation oncologist apologizes for any offense given by his directive not to use the "hair oil" and explains the problem of using oil with dermatitis on the scalp. Together, they negotiate a plan to use the oil only on the chest, back, abdomen, and the part of the head not affected by the dermatitis. Both the family and the oncologist will inspect Mr. Chaudhry's scalp regularly to see if dermatitis has spread.

Multiple attempts to address advance directives with the son have been unsuccessful. The son wishes his father to be a full code. He believes his father will be cured and that his outcome is in Allah's hands. He gets angry with the doctors and thinks they just want to get rid of his father because they want to save money. The palliative care team in the hospital is consulted, and they obtain an interpreter who is not related to the patient. The interview with Mr. Chaudhry is conducted at a time when family is not present. During the interview, the patient starts to cry and says multiple times that he wishes he were dead. He says he is so ashamed of the fact that he can't walk and that his daughter-in-law has to help him get in and out of bed. He is even more ashamed about the fecal and urinary incontinence and that his daughter-in-law has to see him naked and clean him. He says nothing can be worse than this. He also feels ashamed of the despair he feels and wants to be strong and supportive for his family. He does not want to share his thoughts with his family, because he does not want them to think of him as a weak person. He still defers all decisions regarding his health care to his oldest son, but he wishes that the son would give up and face the reality that he is dying and let him die in peace.

Question:
1. How would you approach the son regarding patient's wishes?

You arrange a family conference and ask a Pakistani male physician to be present during the conference. You ask the patient's permission to have the conference without him, and he agrees and gives you permission to share his feelings with the family.

You tell the family about the patient's wishes and discuss his prognosis. After a long discussion, the family agrees to get hospice care for the patient and take him home. The hospice agency arranges for a male personal care worker to assist with bathing. The family also arranges for a male relative to come and live with them who can provide personal assistance to the patient.

| CASE STUDY **2** | **Too Much Information** |

Objectives

1. Explain the importance of establishing an understanding with patients and families about how clinical information is to be communicated and with whom.
2. Understand the possibility of significant misunderstanding of clinical information that is based on cultural perceptions or lack of English proficiency or both.

Mrs. Aslam is an 85-year-old Pakistani who has been living in North America for past 10 years. She lives with her daughter, Mrs. Sheikh, and her family, and she comes to see the doctor only when she feels she needs to. She enjoys very good health and is very proud of the fact that she has normal blood pressure and has never been admitted to the hospital other than for childbirth (she has six children, all of whom live in the United States). She can speak English but lets her daughter do most of the talking. Mrs. Sheikh brought her to the clinic because she has been looking more tired and has not been cooking regularly. The patient agrees that she feels more tired than usual but attributes it to old age. Upon further questioning, she says that she has been having more pain in her joints and has been taking a "pain killer" to help with it. Mrs. Sheikh informs you that she has bought ibuprofen for her mother in the past and notes that she has been going through the bottle rather rapidly these days. You obtain blood work and schedule another appointment for her in 2 weeks.

Blood test results show severe anemia, with a hemoglobin of 8, and you call the patient at home. Mrs. Aslam answers the phone and informs you that her daughter is not home and that you should call back later. You have a very busy clinic day ahead of you, and since the patient understands English perfectly, you go ahead and tell her the test results anyway. She gets very alarmed and asks you how she could have developed this anemia; she goes on to ask you if this is due to cancer.

You tell her that there are several possibilities for this and that most probably her anemia is due to blood loss secondary to her use of ibuprofen, but that cancer cannot be ruled out. You tell the patient to stop taking ibuprofen and that you would like her to come back to the clinic so that you can examine her further and schedule for her to see a gastroenterologist immediately for possible upper and lower endoscopy. You also discuss the possibility of a blood transfusion. Mrs. Aslam is very polite on the phone and tells you that she has understood everything and will follow up.

Two days later, Mrs. Sheikh calls you very upset and wants to know what you told her mother, because she has been crying and has not gotten out of the bed. She is refusing food and keeps saying that she knows she is dying because the doctor told her that she has cancer and needs emergency procedures.

Question:
1. What went wrong with the communication?

After you explain your findings and recommendations to the daughter, she is calmer but tells you that hereafter you should talk to her first before giving any information to her mother.

Question:
1. How could you have prevented Mrs. Aslam's misunderstanding?

In the initial interaction, the fact that Mrs. Sheikh did most of the talking could have alerted you to the possibility that Mrs. Aslam may not have been comfortable with discussing clinical information. You might have engaged her directly in more conversation to assess her English proficiency and understanding of clinical terms. If you had asked her directly about her perception of her condition, her suspicion and fear of cancer might have emerged, and you would have been able to reassure her. When you made the phone call and talked with Mrs. Aslam, she became alarmed at the information you were giving her and asked about the possibility of cancer. That could have alerted you to the fear that she was feeling. Several options would have been possible at that point: You could have tried to reassure her even more clearly on the phone that there is no evidence at this point that cancer is present and emphasize again that the most probable cause of the anemia is the ibuprofen. Or, knowing that in the Pakistani culture family members are often involved with health care decisions of elders, you could have called back later that evening to talk to Mrs. Sheikh to explain the information you had given Mrs. Aslam and your recommendations. For yet another alternative, you could have asked Mrs. Aslam to come in the next day, preferably with her daughter, to be sure you could follow up quickly to diagnose and treat her anemia and also reduce her fear of cancer and death.

References

Ahmad J, Qadeer A. *Science of Graeco-Arabic Medicine.* New Delhi, India: Hamdard University Press; 1998.

Athar S. *Health Concerns for Believers: Contemporary Issues.* Chicago: Kazi Publications; 1996.

Athar S. Information for health care providers when dealing with a Muslim patient. Islamic Medical Association of North America; 1998. Available at: www.imana.org/mc/page.do?sitePageId=7719 (accessed November 2005).

Bender KG. Social problems in Pakistani psychiatric patients. *Int J Soc Psychiatry* 2001;47(3)32–41.

Bhopal R, Unwin N, White M, et al. Heterogeneity of coronary heart disease risk factors in Indian, Pakistani, Bangladeshi, and European origin populations: cross sectional study. *BMJ* 1999;319(7204):215–220.

Gatrad R, Sheikh A. Palliative care for Muslims and issues after death. *Int J Palliat Nurs* 2002;8(12):594–597.

Hunte PA, Sultana F. Health-seeking behavior and the meaning of medications in Balochistan, Pakistan. *Soc Sci Med* 1992;34(12):1385–1397.

Husain N, Creed F, Tomensen B. Adverse social circumstances and depression in people of Pakistani origin in the UK. *Br J Psychiatry* 1997;171:434–438.

Husain N, Creed F, Tomensen B. Depression and social stress in Pakistan. *Psychol Med* 2000;30(2):395–402.

Jan R, Smith CA. Staying healthy in immigrant Pakistani families living in the United States. *J Nurs Scholarsh* 1998;30(2):157–159.

Kamath SK, Murillo G. Breast cancer risk factors in two distinct ethnic groups: Indian and Pakistani vs. American premenopausal women. *Nutr Cancer* 1999;35(1):16–26.

Khan I, Pillay K. User's attitude towards home and hospital treatment: a comparative study between South Asian and white residents of the British Isles. *J Psychiatr Ment Health Nurs* 2000;10(2):137.

Kleinman, A. Culture, illness and cure: clinical lessons from anthropologic and cross-cultural research. *Ann Int Med* 1978;88:251–258.

Low DA, Brasted H. *Freedom, Trauma, Continuities: Northern India and Independence*. Studies on South Asia; vol. 2. Walnut Creek, CA: AltaMira Press (Sage Publications); 1998.

Maher R, Lee AJ, Warnakulasuriya KA, et al. Role of areca nut in the causation of oral submucous fibrosis: a case-control study in Pakistan. *J Oral Pathol Med* 1994;23(2):65–69.

Mull JD, Mull DS. Mothers' concepts of childhood diarrhea in rural Pakistan: what ORT program planners should know. *Soc Sci Med* 1988;27(1):53–67.

Mull JD, Wood CS, Gans LP, et al. Culture and compliance among leprosy patients in Pakistan. *Soc Sci Med* 1989;29(7):799–811.

Pappas G, Akhtar T, Gergen P, et al. Health status of Pakistani population: a health profile and comparison with the United States. *Am J Public Health* 2001;91(1):93–98.

Smith JI. *Islam in America.* New York: Columbia University Press; 1999.

Vickers A, Zollman C. ABC of complementary medicine: homeopathy. *BMJ* 1999;319:1115–1118.

Yeo G, Hikoyeda N. Asian and Pacific Islander elders. In: Maddox G, ed. *Encyclopedia of Aging.* 4th ed. New York: Springer, 2006.

Young JJ, Gu N. *Demographic and Socio-economic Characteristics of Elderly Asian and Pacific Island Americans.* Seattle: National Asian Pacific Center on Aging; 1995.

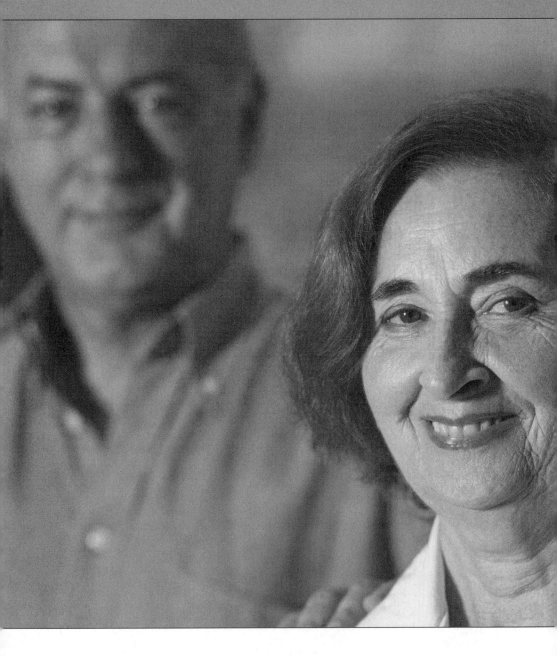

CHAPTER 8

Older Portuguese Americans

Doorway Thoughts

The modest and quiet Portuguese community has captured little attention from the larger American society, as is evident by the lack of literature on the Portuguese immigrants.

Typical older Portuguese immigrants have a calm, resolute approach to their personal medical needs. As dictated by tradition, their youth was likely to have been filled with care-taking activities for the whole family, and in their old age they await their turn in receiving comfort and direction from both their families and their medical providers. The culturally competent clinician working with this ethnic group is advised to remain attentive to their personal opinions and wishes while offering health care expertise.

> *Typical older Portuguese immigrants have a calm, resolute approach to their personal medical needs.*

Preferred Cultural Terms

Portuguese Americans or simply *Portuguese* are accepted terms to refer to this ethnic group. Because of their strong geographical and political roots, some individuals may prefer to be recognized as someone from the mainland in Europe—Continental—or as an islander—Azorean. Immigrants from Madeira are few; it is considered respectful to acknowledge their unique origins.

Formality of Address

Older Portuguese immigrants were socialized at a time and in a culture where respect for authority figures and for elders was the norm. In a professional encounter, Portuguese elders recognize the high status of the medical provider by addressing him or her as *Doutor(a)* or *Senhor(a)*. In this tradition, authority figures are not to be questioned, and the interactive style of Portuguese

American elders may be humble and formal; that is, they may ask a minimal number of questions and seldom dispute or even question diagnosis and treatment options.

In turn, Portuguese American elders—regardless of their social class—will most likely expect to be treated with the consideration and respect that their age merits. Clinicians are advised to start with a formal but friendly attitude in the clinical encounter. This means offering a greeting that is warm but not invasive, giving a handshake, addressing patients either by their first or last names, but always preceding these with *Senhor* ("mister") or *Senhora* or *Dona* ("lady"). Acculturation has led many immigrants to use the more familiar form of the word "you"—*tu*—to communicate with others even in more formal social interactions. If the clinician is speaking in Portuguese, it is still most appropriate to address a Portuguese American elder with the third-person polite pronoun *você*.

> *Clinicians are advised to start with a formal but friendly attitude in the clinical encounter.*

Attitudes Toward North American Health Services

Older Portuguese Americans may expect a holistic approach in their medical care, and a culturally sensitive clinician not only will ask questions and perform examinations directed at diagnosis but also will take the time to ask questions about patients' general well-being and their interactions with the immediate family. By taking care to demonstrate a genuine personal interest in the patient, the clinician may establish solid rapport and trust in the clinical encounter. Such interactions may include tactful exploration of the possible stresses in the patient's personal life that may be hindering the ability to heal, such as a lack of financial resources, isolation, or depression or anxiety.

Older Portuguese American immigrants lived in Portugal when the country was ruled by dictatorial politics and profound traditional Catholic beliefs. Strict political, religious, and social regulations were enforced mainly through fear and public shame. Social expression and activism were frowned upon. As a result, older Portuguese American immigrants

> *Older Portuguese American immigrants may be friendly but also reserved and cautious with outsiders.*

may be friendly but also reserved and cautious with outsiders. This may also be true in medical encounters, where communication may improve as familiarity and trust are built over time.

Language Literacy

One language, Portuguese, is spoken in Portugal, with accents and idiomatic expressions varying by region. Some accents—for example, the one from Saint Michael Island in the Azores—may pose a challenge to nonnative speakers. Similarly, patients may report difficulty in understanding providers and interpreters who speak Portuguese with an accent from a region or country (e.g., Brazil) not their own. In a professional encounter between Portuguese speakers, it is advisable to avoid miscommunication by taking the time to review patients' understanding of the clinical discussion. An advisable technique in such scenarios would be to ask the patient to describe in his or her own words the salient issues being discussed.

Although many older Portuguese immigrants are fluent in English, a significant number of them have little or no command of the language. Just like most individuals for whom English is the second language, it is possible that under stress, patients may feel more comfortable speaking Portuguese, and they may ask for an interpreter during clinical encounters. Most American-born Portuguese elders are fluent in English and acculturated to American social norms.

Respectful Nonverbal Communication

For older Portuguese Americans, respectful nonverbal communication with health care providers starts before they meet. Customarily, patients will bathe and dress themselves in their best clothes to go to a health care appointment. Similarly, they may expect their providers to dress in conservative, good-quality attire that conveys the importance of their status.

Portuguese elders regard the people who take care of their medical needs as part of their most immediate support group, and consequently they may become more intimate with them. Formal greetings in the Portuguese culture in-

They may expect their providers to dress in conservative, good quality attire that conveys the importance of their status.

By resisting these public displays of respectful affection, the clinician may risk appearing unnecessarily aloof or impersonal.

volve direct eye contact and handshakes, even between the sexes, and close relationships invariably involve hugs and two kisses, one on each cheek. If comfortable with this practice, a clinician may accept a hug or a kiss on the cheek from a thankful patient, usually an older woman. In fact, by resisting these public displays of respectful affection, the clinician may risk appearing unnecessarily aloof or impersonal. The use of a formal but open demeanor, mixed with good common sense, is advised in such encounters with Portuguese elders.

Elephants in the Room

Most Portuguese elders prefer Portuguese-speaking providers who also understand their culture. However, there are a very limited number of professionals who meet these requirements.

The concept of preventive medicine is a relatively new one for Portuguese elders. Traditionally, they would seek medical care for acute conditions only. They may also view screening tests with suspicion, because they may associate these tests with the diagnosis of serious illnesses such as cancer.

Providers are viewed as knowledgeable and caring authority figures who should give their professional advice regarding the plan of treatment. Although patients will eventually decide for themselves whether to comply with that plan, they tend to dislike being asked to make important decisions without their providers' guidance.

Among Portuguese American elders, there is a general perception that if a problem requires a medical visit, then it should also warrant a prescription; it may therefore be disappointing if no prescription or only an over-the-counter medication is recommended for an acute problem. It is recommended that the clinician be proactive in spending some time educating older Portuguese patients regarding the utility and limitations of using pharmaceuticals for all health problems. For instance, instead of just recommending conservative treatment for a viral illness, the clinician might give the patient an explanation, such as the immediate undesirable side effects of antibiotics and dangers of drug resistance, while also validating their concerns.

Mental illness carries some stigma in the Portuguese culture, so it is common for older Portuguese Americans to associate their symptoms only with somatic problems and to discuss with the clinician only physical (i.e., medical) complaints. The astute clinician will therefore remain alert for presentations that suggest an underlying mental health concern, particularly when multiple somatic complaints are present or symptoms do not readily lead to another diagnosis.

Among Portuguese American elders, there is a general perception that if a problem requires a medical visit, then it should also warrant a prescription.

In the Portuguese culture, wine is often attributed with invigorating power, and some older Portuguese patients may be reluctant to discontinue its use even if it interacts with their medications. When advised to avoid the use of alcohol, some patients may continue drinking their wine without admitting to providers that they are not following instructions. The culturally sensitive clinician will incorporate patients' beliefs into care planning in order to reach appropriate compromises and achieve optimal clinical efficacy.

Money is another sensitive issue. Older Portuguese Americans are very private about their personal finances and view with some suspicion inquiries that require them to disclose this information. This may have an impact on several health care issues, such as applying for medication coverage, health insurance, or assistance programs.

History of Immigration

Portuguese explorers were among the leading explorers in the 15th century and were the first Europeans to discover and map California. Small Portuguese Jewish communities were established in North America in the 1600s, and a Portuguese colony was established in what is now Hawaii in the 1700s.

The first period of Portuguese mass immigration occurred between about 1870 and 1920, mainly from the Azores, to the locations where the earliest Portuguese settlements had been established: southeastern New England, central California, and Hawaii. After a dormant period, mass Portuguese immigration resumed in 1958 following a volcanic eruption in the Azores island of Faial. Portuguese immigration to the United States virtually ended in the 1980s after peaking in the 1970s. During this period Portuguese immigrants settled in Massachusetts, New Jersey, Rhode Island, and Connecticut.

Degree of Acculturation

As with all immigrant groups, the degree of acculturation of Portuguese American individuals varies widely. To avoid stereotyping, the culturally astute clinician will inquire about each person's cultural preferences and attitudes.

At the time that older Portuguese immigrants were growing up in Portugal, only a fourth-grade education was mandatory. The vast majority of Portuguese immigrants were from poor rural areas, where parents counted on children to contribute to the family welfare either with labor or by performing household tasks. As a consequence, many Portuguese children frequently missed school, resulting in very low levels of literacy in Portuguese.

Upon their arrival in the United States, this older generation's main concern was financial stability for the family; consequently, education was less valued than work. The Portuguese immigrants usually worked long hours in factories, cleaning jobs, agriculture, and the service industries, leaving little time for English classes. The motivation to learn English was further hindered by the fact that most Portuguese immigrants worked with other immigrants and lived in Portuguese-speaking neighborhoods that could meet their social and community needs. Even when not fully acculturated to mainstream society, older Portuguese Americans may nevertheless say that they have been successful in accomplishing their dream of social and financial upward mobility.

Following in the footsteps of their parents, Portuguese immigrants in the 1970s often allowed their children to drop out of school at age 16 in order to start working and contributing to the family's maintenance and future financial security. Children often assumed responsibility and authority for language translation for the family, a role that could provoke conflict if parents felt disrespected. Today, in spite of the availability of interpretive services in many hospitals and clinics, some older Portuguese Americans have grown accustomed to having their children take them to the doctor and help make health decisions for them. Although generally caring and dutiful in this caretaking role, the acculturated children of Portuguese immigrants at times report feeling burdened by having to assume multiple responsibilities (e.g., driving, interpreting, translating, getting information, and helping to make informed decisions) for their parents.

Tradition and Health Beliefs

The authors' medical and mental health clinical experiences have alerted them to the possibility that Portuguese immigrants may hide nonadherence with Western biomedical treatments (e.g., changing dosages, no longer taking medications, not following prescribed diets) and instead use alternatives that include herbal therapies recommended by *curandeiros* (traditional healers). Traditional healers are lay people who, through informal training or by their own ability, have gained community recognition for their healing gift. Some of their practices involve making predictions by using clients' personal objects or special books and cards. The healers may also evoke or send away harmful spirits, especially *mau olhado* (devil's eye). Another type of popular healer is the *endireita,* an individual who uses the bare hands to repair sprained joints and muscles. In addition, many older Portuguese Americans are devout Roman Catholics, and they may rely on receiving healing grace from a patron saint or the Holy Spirit.

Traditional healers are lay people who, through informal training or by their own ability, have gained community recognition for their healing gift.

Older Portuguese Americans may be resistant to referrals for mental health care, in the belief that obtaining these services entails being labeled as "crazy." The stigma associated with mental health care results largely from past experience in Portugal, where mental health services are mostly restricted to major mental illness. Being *nervoso(a)* (nervous) is the usual expression they use to refer to their psychological distress and work- or family-related stress.

Culture-Specific Health Risks

Very little has been published regarding health risks specific to the Portuguese American community. A study done by the Cambridge Health Alliance in the Massachusetts cities of Cambridge and Somerville revealed that Portuguese patients are less likely than the general public to receive screening tests such as mammograms and colonoscopies. These results are similar to known data pertaining to other minority groups.

No studies have been done regarding either the incidence or prevalence of specific disease conditions in Portuguese Americans. In our professional practice with Portuguese elders, we encounter multiple cases of diabetes mellitus, heart disease, hyperlipidemia, and obesity. Smoking and related illnesses such as chronic obstructive pulmonary disease are quite prevalent, particularly among older men, who may have started smoking in their early teens. Alcohol, more specifically red wine, is a traditional component of the Portuguese diet, and it is not uncommon for patients to drink one or two glasses of wine with meals. A thorough history is essential to detect possible alcohol overuse or abuse.

> *Alcohol, more specifically red wine, is a traditional component of the Portuguese diet, and it is not uncommon for patients to drink one or two glasses of wine with meals.*

Approaches to Decision Making

Family has a central and essential role for many older Portuguese patients. Relatives, and especially daughters and sons, are commonly expected to take care of their older parents. As such, nursing-home placement may be associated with feelings of abandonment by the elders and of guilt by their families. It is quite common for older Portuguese patients to defer decisions pertaining to their health to their children. A possible explanation for this attitude is their awareness of changes in science and their inability to keep up with them. They believe and trust their children's knowledge and feel that the younger people are better equipped to make these decisions.

> *They believe and trust their children's knowledge and feel that the younger people are better equipped to make these decisions.*

Attitudes Regarding Disclosure and Consent

Portuguese people may avoid discussing death, feeling that it may come their way by just mentioning it. In traditional Portuguese culture, serious or terminal diagnosis would be hidden from the patient and disclosed only to family members. American Portuguese families may be shocked when a clinician tells the patient directly of a diagnosis and prognosis. When delivering bad news to an older Portuguese American patient, it is very important to set aside sufficient time for a full and holistic conversation. Simple explanations are advisable; eliciting feedback from patients (or their appointed decision makers) is an excellent way to confirm their understanding of the information. Nodding and simple words of agreement are not necessarily signs that the message has been understood; some older patients may have been educated not to disagree with authority figures. It is also important to be attentive to each patient's wishes by asking what he or she would like to know about the disease and to revisit the question at subsequent visits.

To learn the current disclosure preferences of Portuguese American elders, the authors surveyed people at one Portuguese senior day center. Of the 53 people interviewed (26 men and 27 women), the majority wanted to be told about a life-threatening diagnosis; half of them also wanted their families to be part of the disclosure. The majority of the elders preferred to be included in the medical providers' discussions of treatment. Although the information from this informal survey cannot be generalized, it supported our impression that most Portuguese elders want to be involved in their health care decisions and that a large number of them also want their families involved.

Gender Issues

For older Portuguese Americans, changes in gender roles were largely precipitated by immigration. Brought up in a patriarchal society, Portuguese men were the authority figure in and the financial providers for the family; women were the caretakers in charge of the home, children, and sick elders and commonly were also their husbands' helpers in farming. Regardless of their status in the family, wives generally deferred to their husbands. In the United States, however, many Portuguese American women entered the

In general, older Portuguese women are more receptive than men to treatments, both medical and psychological.

workforce, thereby gaining financial independence that led to a more equal status with men in their families and communities.

In general, older Portuguese women are more receptive than men to treatments, both medical and psychological. Portuguese American elders may be more comfortable with same-sex providers, although this factor may become less important if there is a strong bond between the patient and the clinician. Past cultural norms valued female modesty, so it is common for older Portuguese women to decline routine gynecologic care; it may require extra effort to convince them of its importance.

End-of-Life Decision Making and Care Intensity

Portuguese Americans generally rely heavily on the input of family and clinicians regarding end-of-life decisions. Religion also

Being predominantly Roman Catholic, older Portuguese Americans may favor do-not-resuscitate orders as being the same as "following God's wishes."

plays a significant role. Being predominantly Roman Catholic, older Portuguese Americans may favor do-not-resuscitate (DNR) orders as being the same as "following God's wishes." For example, the majority of elders interviewed at the previously mentioned Portuguese senior center revealed a determination not to be resuscitated. However, it is common for family members to disagree and to equate DNR orders with neglectful care. As with many cultural groups and individuals, it may be important in working with Portuguese elders, therefore, to clarify the exact meaning of a DNR order and to assure the elder and family members that the elder will receive comprehensive care, short of cardiopulmonary resuscitation, if such an order is signed.

For terminal care, the elders at the Portuguese senior center indicated a desire to stay in their home environment. The majority of them preferred to be treated in their own home and to go to a hospital only when intensive care was necessary. Unquestionably, living in a nursing home or in a relative's home was not preferred for terminal care.

Use of Advance Directives

It is not customary for older Portuguese Americans to discuss death and dying, and it is common for them to delay conversations about the topic until they are acutely ill. It is advisable to introduce the topic carefully over several visits and to schedule a meeting with the patient and selected family members so that enough time can be given to the discussion of advance directives and all their questions and concerns can be addressed.

It is common for Portuguese patients not to have a clear code status at time of hospitalization. In our interviews at the senior center, we found that only 10 out of 53 individuals had assigned a proxy for health decisions, although the majority of these seniors also stated that they had a person (customarily a spouse or adult child) to make their medical decisions if they became incapacitated. However, seniors also reported that conversations on such matters had not necessarily taken place among important family members as a group. The culturally sensitive clinician will be alert to these issues and diplomatically encourage their Portuguese American patients to clarify their wishes with their closest family members and with key clinicians well in advance of critical clinical situations.

It is common for Portuguese patients not to have a clear code status at time of hospitalization.

Ana Perry Nava, PhD
Helena Santos-Martins, MD

| CASE STUDY **1** | **Cancer Is a Scary Word** |

Objectives

1. Examine the ways that taboos related to screening tests affect the health of Portuguese American elders.
2. Understand the need to respect the patient's choice not to know a terminal diagnosis.
3. Understand family's role in patient care.
4. Understand the role of the primary care physician in safeguarding the patient's wishes while navigating the medical system.
5. Explore ways to respect taboos in the Portuguese culture usually associated with the words *cancer* and *biopsy*.

Mr. Mario Medeiros is an 82-year-old man from the island of Saint Michael, Azores. He immigrated to the United States over 30 years ago and speaks only Portuguese. He lives with his wife on the first floor of a two-family house. One of his three daughters lives on the top floor with her family. She and her other sisters check on their parents daily and frequently share meals with them. Mr. Medeiros has been relatively healthy for his age, with hypertension and coronary heart disease, both well-controlled.

Dr. Sofia Oliveira is a 45-year-old internist who is bilingual in Portuguese. She is well-acquainted with the Portuguese culture, because she was born in Portugal and has lived in the United States for over 20 years. She practices in the public health system in a neighborhood clinic near Mr. Medeiros' home. She has been his primary care physician for 10 years, and they have a solid patient-doctor relationship.

Mr. Medeiros has been very diligent in attending his routine follow-up appointments, but he has consistently declined routine screening tests, such as digital rectal examinations and colonoscopy. He usually comes to his appointments alone.

One day, Mr. Medeiros comes to the clinic for a sick visit, accompanied by his wife and their three daughters. The women are very concerned about an "ulcer" Mrs. Medeiros noticed in the patient's perirectal area while she was helping him with his personal hygiene. It has been worsening and now has started to bleed. Mr. Medeiros had dismissed their previous concerns and declined to seek medical attention. After much convincing, they were now able to bring him to see Dr. Oliveira.

Dr. Oliveira obtains the history from the patient, his wife, and their daughters, but also wishes to perform an examination alone with the patient and a nurse chaperone. The patient looks younger than his age, he is pleasant and well groomed, and he is in no apparent distress. He agrees to the rectal examination. Dr. Oliveira finds a large fungating mass with ulcerated areas in the external rectal area, highly suspicious for a rectal malignancy.

Question:
1. How would you explain your concerns about the diagnosis to the patient?

Dr. Oliveira asks Mr. Medeiros if he has any idea what the problem is, and he replies that he really doesn't want to know. He thinks that probably it is "not good," and he trusts Dr. Oliveira to do and recommend what it is best for him. He will follow Dr. Oliveira's advice, but he says he doesn't want to know the diagnosis. He gives permission to have the daughters and the wife involved in the discussion.

Question:
1. How might Dr. Oliveira be certain that the patient gets the treatment and family support that he needs?

Dr. Oliveira asks the daughters and Mrs. Medeiros to return to the room and reports that the "ulcer" needs specialized treatment. She refers Mr. Medeiros to general surgery for "further tests," and she avoids using the word *biopsy,* because she knows it is usually associated with a malignancy in the Portuguese culture. While the patient is making the appointment, two of the daughters and wife stay behind and ask to speak privately with Dr. Oliveira.

Question:
1. How best can Dr. Oliveira convey the patient's likely diagnosis to his daughters and wife?

Dr. Oliveira explains to them her concern for malignancy, which the daughters admit to having suspected already. They also inform Dr. Oliveira that Mr. Medeiros will never want to know the true diagnosis, in the event that a cancer is confirmed. Dr. Oliveira calls the surgeon and notifies him of the patient's wishes.

A biopsy confirms anal cancer, further work-up reveals extensive colon involvement, and the patient is referred to a tertiary care center for evaluation. Despite undergoing radiation and chemotherapy, Mr. Medeiros' health starts to decline quite rapidly.

Two months later he is seen in follow-up for his hypertension by Dr. Oliveira, who again asks him about his current understanding of his condition. Mr. Medeiros states that the "ulcer" is causing him a lot of pain, but he feels much better with the pain medications. He goes on to say that he "knows" that it is "not good" but that he is "in God's hands." He also tells Dr. Oliveira that it is really important for him to stay at home and not be sent to a nursing home.

Mr. Medeiros is referred to a home hospice program. He dies peacefully at home 2 months later, surrounded by his family.

| CASE STUDY **2** | **Forever a Mother** |

Objectives
1. Understand the importance of collaboration between medical and mental health providers.
2. Understand how the role of being a mother, in the Portuguese culture, may be given priority over self-care needs.

Mrs. Manuela Ferreira is a 66-year-old Portuguese woman who presents to her doctor with a 5-day history of progressive left ankle and foot pain with swelling since a fall at home the previous week. Mrs. Ferreira is a widow and the sole caretaker of her adult mentally retarded daughter. She is also very protective of her and her family's privacy, having declined various types of professional help in the past, such as home care services.

Mrs. Ferreira's primary care physician for the past 2 years is Dr. Armando Silva, a 50-year-old bilingual and bicultural internist with a large geriatrics practice who has been practicing in the same neighborhood clinic for about 15 years. She had transferred care to him from a larger clinic at the advice of her longtime bilingual psychotherapist, Dr. Madalena Sousa, who was concerned about the lack of optimal communication between Mrs. Ferreira and her former American providers (Mrs. Ferreira only had limited English skills and interpreters were not always available). Dr. Sousa, who had an in-depth knowledge of the Portuguese culture, also wanted to facilitate better communication among the mental and medical providers, because coordination of care in Mrs. Ferreira's case was of utmost importance, given the complexity of her psychological and medical histories. These included difficult-to-control chronic depression with psychotic episodes, uncontrolled diabetes mellitus with neuropathy, coronary heart disease, hyperlipidemia, and hypertension. Since transferring to Dr. Silva, Mrs. Ferreira's overall status had gradually improved, and she had been stable for the past year.

When Dr. Silva enters the examining room, he finds Mrs. Ferreira in obvious discomfort. He has to help her to get up on the examining table because she is limping and unable to bear weight on her left foot. Mrs. Ferreira is apologetic and reports having delayed obtaining medical care for her ankle because she hoped she would get better on her own; she needed to continue performing her household chores and taking care of her daughter. Mrs. Ferreira proceeds to emphasize how important it is for her to be her daughter's caretaker, as she firmly believes that, being the mother, she is the only person who can give the love and attention her daughter requires. On examination, her left foot is found to be edematous, with point tenderness and highly suspicious for an ankle fracture.

Questions:
1. How should Dr. Silva interpret Mrs. Ferreira's delay in seeking medical care?
2. How can he best convey to her the high likelihood of a fracture and get her to accept home services?

Dr. Silva is aware of Mrs. Ferreira's vulnerability regarding the stigma of mental illness in the Portuguese community, as well as cultural expectations regarding motherhood. This has been possible because of the ongoing collaboration between Drs. Silva and Sousa in coordinating Mrs. Ferreira's care. For instance, he knows that she has feelings of shame and guilt about her daughter's condition as well as her own struggles with chronic depression; she feels vulnerable to community gossip. As such, she isolates herself despite multiple attempts by Dr. Sousa to convince her to join community programs, such as the local Portuguese senior center.

With this in mind, Dr. Silva tells Mrs. Ferreira that he understands why she did not see him sooner and that he is aware of her responsibilities at home. He also informs her that, given the high likelihood of a fracture, she'll need immediate radiography at the local hospital to confirm the diagnosis. He explains that if indeed she has a fracture, she'll need a cast and will not be able to bear weight on her left foot. He kindly emphasizes to her the need to accept at least temporary help so that her recovery can be complete.

The clinic's secretary arranges for an immediate orthopedic appointment preceded by radiography; she calls a taxi to take Mrs. Ferreira to the hospital. One hour later, Dr. Silva gets a call from the radiology department confirming a nondisplaced fracture of the ankle. The patient is seen in the orthopedics department, where her foot is placed in a cast and she is put on non-weight-bearing status. Arrangements are made that day for a visiting nurse, home safety evaluation, and home physical therapy, which are reluctantly accepted by the patient. Mrs. Ferreira, however, adamantly refuses home visits from the hospital's social worker, as well as home deliveries for meals. She states that she is very careful about her diet because of her diabetes and heart condition, and that she eats only homemade Portuguese food. She has no plan for the care of her daughter.

Question:
1. How can the psychotherapist and the primary care provider help this homebound patient?

Dr. Silva calls Mrs. Ferreira at home later that day. Understanding her responsibilities for taking care of her daughter, the importance of good nutrition, and how difficult it has been to keep her depression under control, Dr. Silva worries that this new situation may trigger a relapse, and he wants to enlist Dr. Sousa's help. With Mrs. Ferreira's permission, he calls Dr. Sousa, who also calls her patient at home.

Dr. Sousa talks extensively with patient about the fracture and the repercussions it has in her life. Together, they develop a comprehensive plan that includes periodic check-in calls by Dr. Sousa to monitor her mental status and daily living conditions. The patient also agrees to have a relative deliver groceries and home-cooked meals and temporarily have her daughter stay with another close family member.

Despite these arrangements, 3 weeks later Mrs. Ferreira starts becoming overwhelmed by her new, albeit temporary disability, and her depression begins to resurface. Concerned that she may decompensate as well as foreseeing future difficulties with her self-care and her ability to care adequately for her mentally retarded daughter, Drs. Sousa and Silva propose a family meeting. Mrs. Ferreira initially resists the idea and insists that she is self-sufficient. Although she is not ready to commit to any permanent changes, she later agrees to the meeting and requests the presence of her two family members who have been very supportive of her. During the meeting, Mrs. Ferreira reiterates that it is very important for her to continue caring for her daughter; otherwise, she will feel that she failed at meeting her motherhood responsibilities, but she now admits to needing more permanent help. Her relatives volunteer their continued support, and Mrs. Ferreira accepts agency home services. Her daughter moves back home.

References

Adler JP. *The Portuguese in Cambridge and Somerville* (combined edition). Cambridge, MA: Cambridge Community Development Department; 1980.

Araujo Z. Portuguese families. In: McGoldrick M, Pearce J, Giordano J, eds. *Ethnicity and Family Therapy*. New York: Guilford Press; 1996:583–594.

Graves AR. *The Portuguese Californians—Immigrants in Agriculture*. San Jose, CA: Portuguese Heritage Publications of California, Inc.; 2004.

James S. Agonias: the social and sacred suffering of Azorean immigrants. *Cult Med Psychiatry* 2002;26:87–110.

Mira M. *The Forgotten Portuguese—The Melungeons and Other Groups: The Portuguese Making of America*. Franklin, NC: The Portuguese-American Historical Research Foundation, Inc.; 1998.

Moitosa E. Portuguese families. In: McGoldrick M, Pearce J, Giordano J, eds. *Ethnicity and Family Therapy*. New York: Guilford Press; 1982:412–437.

Nava A. *Acculturation to Psychotherapy: The Experience of Portuguese and Brazilian Immigrant Women in the U.S.A.* [dissertation]. Boston, MA: Simmons College School of Social Work; 2000.

Pap L. *The Portuguese-Americans*. 2nd ed. Boston, MA: Portuguese Continental Union of the USA; 1992.

Simas RMN, ed. *Women in the Azores and the Immigrant Communities*. São Miguel, Azores: EGA–Empresa Gráfica Açoreana, Lda.; 2003.

CHAPTER 9

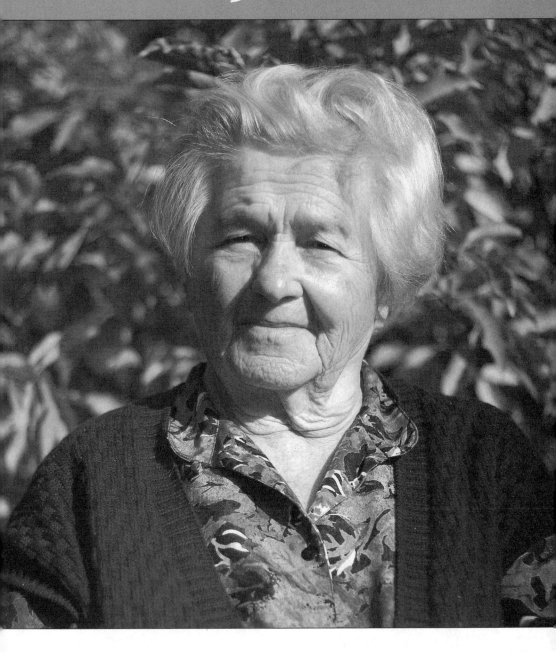

Older Russian-Speaking Americans

Preferred Cultural Terms

In the United States, the term *Russian immigrant* is widely used. The preferred term, however, is *Russian-speaking immigrant*. The former Soviet Union was a conglomerate of many former nations that included not only Russia, but also Ukraine, Armenia, Byelorussia, and many others. Most of the people who left the former Soviet Union are not of Russian heritage and were not considered Russian when they resided there. Rather, their religious heritage is most commonly Jewish, but they may also be Armenian or Ukrainian, for example. What unites these people today is the Russian language.

Some immigrants from the former Soviet Union are offended by being identified as Russian in the United States, because the Soviet government marginalized their heritage, forcing them to adopt the Russian language and culture. Referring to this immigrant group as Russian-speaking rather than Russian is not only technically more correct but also minimizes the risk of causing offense.

Formality of Address

It is permissible to address older Russian-speaking Americans as Mr. or Mrs. when first meeting them. However, older Russian speakers may wish to establish a personal relationship with their health providers and may interpret being called by their first name in subsequent clinical encounters as a sign that the relationship has become more personal. Of note is that the patronymic, not the last name, is part of formal address in the Russian language. For example, if the patient's name is Vladimir Sergeeovich Melnychuk (literally meaning, Vladimir Melnychuk, son of Sergei), his colleagues but not his family or close friends

Some immigrants from the former Soviet Union are offended by being identified as Russian in the United States.

would formally refer to him as Vladimir Sergeeovich. Likewise, if his daughter is named Irina, her name will be Irina Vladimirovna Melnychuk (i.e., Irina, daughter of Vladimir), and her colleagues but not her family or close friends would formally refer to her as Irina Vladimirovna.

Respectful Nonverbal Communication

In a clinical encounter with a Russian-speaking elder, it is recommended that clinicians make eye contact, smile, and communicate that they are genuinely interested. Spending time listening will most likely be very important, and taking phone calls or checking one's watch will most likely be considered rude or uncaring. In addition, older Russian-speaking Americans will commonly expect to speak directly to their clinician and may be greatly upset if they are not able to do so when they telephone for advice.

History of Immigration

Russian-speaking Americans are from the former Soviet Union or one of the post-Soviet independent states, including Russia, Armenia, Ukraine, Moldova, Georgia, Azerbaijan, Belarus, Uzbekistan, Kyrgyzstan, Kazakhstan, Turkmenistan, Tajikistan, Lithuania, Latvia, and Estonia. Contemporary immigration began in the 1970s, when the United States granted refugee status to religious and ethnic minorities because of their persecution by the Soviet government. Soviet Jews were the largest ethnic-religious minority, followed by Soviet Armenians, Pentecostals, and Evangelicals. After the dissolution of the Soviet Union in 1991, Russian-speaking immigrants were given the opportunity by their government to emigrate as nonrefugees. These post-Soviet immigrants included some ethnic Russians who left mostly for economic reasons. The majority of these later immigrants, however, continued to be ethnic and religious minorities who came to the United States with refugee status.

Most Russian-speaking immigrants are highly educated and were professionals in their homeland.

Most Russian-speaking immigrants are highly educated and were professionals in their homeland. For example, one in six was a scientist, engineer, or medical doctor. Unlike many other immigrant groups, a large proportion of people came as extended families, bringing elderly family members with them.

Degree of Acculturation

The degree of acculturation is typically low for elders but higher for their children. Most Russian-speaking Americans are concentrated in ethnic enclaves in certain cities in the United States, such as New York, San Francisco, Boston, and Chicago, where they have their own media (radio, newspapers, and television) and grocery stores. Older Russian-speaking Americans tend to live in elder housing with other Russian-speaking elders. Therefore, they also tend to interact mainly with others who share their same language and culture.

Language and Literacy

Older Russian-speaking Americans may have limited English-speaking skills, mostly because they emigrated in later life and had no opportunity to learn English by working in the United States. However, most Russian-speaking elders are highly educated, and their education may have included reading professional texts in English. In these instances, their ability to read in English is higher than their ability to speak it. Of note is that a significant number of Russian-speaking American elders were physicians in their homeland. Consequently, literacy with regard to medical terms is high in this subgroup.

Tradition and Health Beliefs

Western biomedicine was the predominant medical approach in the former Soviet Union. Consequently, older Russian-speaking Americans are used to the medical approach used in the United States. Older Russian speakers tend to subscribe to the Western biomedical beliefs that disease is caused by stress, internal defect, or lifestyle. However, in addition to relying on prescription and over-the-counter medications that are common in mainstream medical practice, older Russian speakers may also engage in health practices common in the former Soviet Union, including reliance on fresh

Older Russian speakers tend to subscribe to the Western biomedical beliefs that disease is caused by stress, internal defect, or lifestyle.

air, herbal remedies, food, light exercise, massage, and relaxation therapies to keep healthy and treat health problems. They may also prefer medical specialists to general practitioners and request—as well as expect—aggressive treatment when they are not feeling well. Depending on the level of acculturation, many older Russian-speaking Americans may use prescription medications from their homeland. It is advisable for clinicians to inquire about this practice in order to avoid unwanted drug interactions.

Home Care and Food

Older Russian-speaking Americans grew up in an era of severe food shortages and may, therefore, attach a lot of significance to food. They commonly prefer their own ethnic foods. When they are hospitalized, they may ask relatives to bring them food from home. Their diet may be high in fat and salt, consisting of fatty meats, fried potatoes, and smoked fish. Chicken broth is considered therapeutic for many minor illnesses.

Older Russian-speaking Americans are likely to be in favor of home care and may view it as a means to remain independent and reduce the burden on their adult children. In view of language constraints, they may prefer home-care agencies with Russian-speaking staff and are highly aware of need-based services such as Meals-on-Wheels, homemaker services, and home-health aides. However, Russian-speaking Americans do not view home care as a substitute for hospital care, and elders may expect to be hospitalized when they are ill. Home-based hospice may not be commonly requested, and families may want loved ones to die in a hospital.

Culture-Specific Health Risks

Older Russian-speaking Americans have lived through war, famine, and mass repression. If they are from Ukraine or other industrialized areas, they may have also been exposed to high levels of environmental contaminants and radiation (from, for example, the nuclear power plant disaster at Chernobyl). Their lifestyle commonly includes smoking, being sedentary, and eating a high-fat, high-salt diet. In comparison with the general U.S. population, older Russian-speaking Americans have higher rates of hypertension, cardiac disease, diabetes mellitus, cancer, and gastrointestinal problems. Many older Russian-speaking Americans also suffer from loneliness, depression, and anxiety, problems that may stem from their past but that are compounded by immigrating to a new culture later in life. Older Russian-speaking Americans are commonly very concerned about their health and may seek health care for minor problems to prevent becoming ill and burdening their families.

> *Many older Russian-speaking Americans also suffer from loneliness, depression, and anxiety.*

Approaches to Decision Making

Older Russian-speaking Americans may have a great reverence for physicians. They and their adult children are likely to expect health providers to be the authority on health matters and to do everything possible to improve their health. Patients and their families commonly assume that clinicians will make the best decisions on their behalf and may interpret efforts to involve them in decisions as an indication that the clinician lacks knowledge and expertise. In view of a common preference for aggressive treatments in this cultural group, even highly educated Russian-speaking Americans may need to be given information on how more aggressive treatment options might affect quality of life. They may not have considered the consequences of more aggressive treatments, mostly because they may not have been exposed to discussions about risk.

Attitudes Regarding Disclosure and Consent

Older Russian-speaking immigrants may become anxious when asked to give informed consent because this is a new experience for them. Obtaining informed consent was not part of medical practice in the former Soviet Union. Children of older Russian-speaking Americans may assume responsibility for obtaining informed consent and disclosing information about their parents' health. According to cultural norms, children may be expected to protect their parents from hearing worrisome news about their health. Therefore, they often describe risks so that they sound less severe or may direct their parents to sign for consent without informing them of the details. Children of older Russian-speaking Americans may also minimize or not disclose diagnoses

According to cultural norms, children may be expected to protect their parents from hearing worrisome news about their health.

that are particularly frightening, such as cancer. The astute clinician may want to use a professional interpreter to ask older Russian-speaking immigrants if they wish to receive information and make their own decisions or wish to include children or other caregivers in decision making. In any event, whenever possible, the skilled provider begins conversations about informed consent by putting risk in a less threatening context, such as by prefacing statements about risk as the worst possible, but not necessarily the most common outcome.

Gender Issues

Older Russian-speaking Americans were reared under the Soviet philosophy of gender equality. Thus, many older Russian-speaking American women were longstanding participants in the Soviet workforce. Their professions included medicine, engineering, and other professions that are not typical for American-born women of comparable age. Nonetheless, there are some gender stereotypes, such as expecting gynecologists to be female and surgeons to be male. Although gender roles in the private sphere are traditional—for example, men's careers take priority over women's and men do not typically perform household chores—both genders are involved in making decisions that affect family life. Men and women's equal participation in decision making includes decisions about health care.

End-of-Life Decision Making and Care Intensity

Older Russian-speaking Americans are not accustomed to discussing issues related to terminal illness and death. In the former Soviet Union, patients and their spouses are not told when an illness is terminal. Cancer, for example, may be perceived by older Russian-speaking Americans as a death sentence, and discussing this diagnosis is commonly taboo. Older Russian-speaking Americans and their families also may not be accustomed to making decisions about end-of-life or palliative care. They are more used to "taking life as it comes" and may perceive planning for death as disrespectful and bad luck. When health providers in the

United States attempt to discuss end-of-life issues, they may be seen as uncaring and taking a too matter-of-fact approach to a highly emotional situation. The sensitive clinician working with this population may wish to present decisions for the end of life after establishing a trusting relationship with the family and in the context of making decisions about quality of life and relieving suffering. Within this context, older Russian-speaking Americans and their adult children may be more likely to be open to the concept of planning for end-of-life care.

> *When health providers in the United States attempt to discuss end-of-life issues, they may be seen as uncaring and taking a too matter-of-fact approach to a highly emotional situation.*

Attitudes Toward Advance Directives

Do-not-resuscitate (DNR) orders, living wills, and health care proxies are rare among older Russian-speaking Americans. Older Russian-speakers and their families commonly have great faith that the Western medical system is capable of curing intractable conditions. As a result, they expect that everything possible will be done to restore health, even in situations where a prognosis is grave. When decisions about advance directives are unavoidable, adult children may wish to assume responsibility. Nonetheless, depending on their level of acculturation, adult children may rely heavily on physicians' advice about advance directives. Adult children may also observe the taboo of not discussing advance directives with their parents.

Elephants in the Room

Older Russian-speaking Americans expect comprehensive health care services and a lot of attention from their health providers, including aggressive medical intervention. They may amplify their health problems in order to get attention and more aggressive medical intervention.

> *Older Russian-speakers and their families commonly have great faith that the Western medical system is capable of curing intractable conditions.*

Older Russian-speaking Americans typically present somatic symptoms as a way of communicating depression or other mental health problems. They avoid mental health practitioners, in part because of the stigma they associate with mental illness, and in part because of prior psychiatric abuses by the Soviet regime as a means of political oppression.

Karen J. Aroian, PhD, RN
Galina Khatutsky, MS
Alexandra Dashevskaya, MA, MS

| CASE STUDY **1** | **Remedies from the Homeland** |

Objective
1. Devise questions for detecting commonly occurring medical problems that result from cultural health practices of Russian-speaking immigrants.

Irina Sobol, a registered nurse, works as a visiting nurse for a large home-care agency in the greater Boston area. She is a first-generation immigrant who speaks fluent Russian; she received her nursing degree in the United States. Irina has a large caseload of homebound older Russian-speaking immigrants who live clustered in one senior housing complex.

Mr. Igor Shorin is one of her regular patients in this senior housing complex, and she sees him weekly for home-health care. He is 87 years old and suffers from heart failure, hypertension, and advanced diabetes mellitus. His ability to perform daily activities of living is very limited because of his health. Mr. Shorin lives with his wife, who is his primary caregiver. He also has two children, who live in the area and visit him regularly.

Irina had taken a diet history when she first started making home-health visits to Mr. Shorin. He prefers traditional Russian foods, including foods high in fat and sodium. His favorite foods are fatty sausages and salty smoked fish. She has told him about how foods high in fat and sodium are not good for his medical condition and has encouraged him to increase his fruit and vegetable intake.

Question:
1. What aspects of Mr. Shorin's diet might be a problem for his medical diagnoses?

Despite Irina's efforts, Mr. Shorin has not changed his diet, and he suffers from severe constipation. After checking his usual prescription medications, Irina calls the doctor to get a standing order for a mild laxative and a stool softener.

Next week when Irina visits Mr. Shorin, she finds him ill and in bed. He is feeling weak and dizzy and is almost unable to walk. His wife reports that he collapsed on his way to the bathroom and could barely get back on his feet. Irina takes his vital signs and begins to ask him a series of questions, trying to understand what is happening.

Question:
1. What questions regarding Mr. Shorin's history regarding medications would be important to ask at this point? Why?

Then she remembers to ask one last question. She knows that her Russian patients tend to self-medicate, so she asks Mr Shorin's wife to list exactly what other prescription and nonprescription medications he might be taking in addition to what is listed in his care plan.

Mrs. Shorin replies that a neighbor, who is also an older Russian-speaking immigrant and was a physician in the former Soviet Union, advised Mrs. Shorin to give her husband a commonly used Russian herbal medication for constipation. Mrs. Shorin dutifully listened to this advice and added the Russian herbal medication to her husband's medication regimen 3 days before Irina's scheduled home visit. It did not occur to Mrs. Shorin that her husband should not take both the Russian herbal and the prescribed medication. As a result of taking the herbal and the prescribed laxatives as well as a stool softener for 3 days, Mr. Shorin has experienced severe diarrhea and dehydration. He needs to be admitted to a local hospital's emergency department to receive intravenous fluids.

| CASE STUDY **2** | **Do Not Talk to Me About It!** |

Objectives

1. Describe the relevant cultural and family values that may preclude an open discussion of end-of-life issues with older Russian-speaking Americans.
2. Devise strategies for providers to introduce and maintain the dialogue with older Russian-speaking Americans and their families to help them understand that end-of-life decisions can affect quality of life and suffering.

Marina Lass is a licensed social worker who was born in Russia but received her training in the United States. She works at a large long-term-care facility and has a caseload of about 50 residents, most of whom are low-income U.S.-born elders on Medicaid. Marina speaks Russian fluently and is accustomed to the American system of counseling and delivering health care.

The registered nurse who processes admissions at the facility asks Marina to get involved in the admission process for an 87-year-old Russian-speaking woman, Dr. Olga Rosenzweig. Dr. Rosenzweig is seeking admission because she lives alone and has limited mobility. She is frail and has suffered multiple bone fractures, including a double hip fracture. She is at risk for future falls and has chronic obstructive pulmonary disease and a chronic heart condition. Despite Dr. Rosenzweig's frail health, she is cognitively intact and very vocal in voicing her opinions. Unlike most residents in this facility, Dr. Rosenzweig is highly educated. Before moving to the United States to join her son, she worked as a physician and practiced internal medicine in Moscow. Her son, also a physician in Moscow, emigrated when he was in the middle of his career. He is now a prospering psychiatrist with an established practice with the local Russian-speaking immigrant community. He states that he feels guilty that he could not have his mother move in with him and care for her, but both he and his mother agree that his work demands would interfere with providing the kind of care she needs.

Dr. Rosenzweig is the first Russian-speaking resident to be admitted to this facility, and she and her son are very excited to discover that there is a Russian-speaking social worker at the facility who can help Dr. Rosenzweig become settled in the facility. Marina is also excited that she has the opportunity to educate Dr. Rosenzweig and her son about the long-term-care system in the United States and can help her adjust to long-term care. As with all admissions, Marina is obligated, within the first 24 hours, to document a new resident's preferences and desires on end-of-life directives, such as whether to resuscitate.

Question:

1. How would you initiate a culturally appropriate discussion of the end-of-life issues that would be both sensitive to Dr. Rosenzweig's cultural background and in compliance with the facility's regulations?

Knowing that end-of-life issues are difficult and not commonly discussed in the Russian-speaking culture, Marina starts the discussion with Dr. Rosenzweig and her son by first inquiring about whether they are familiar with success rates and consequences of performing cardiopulmonary resuscitation (CPR) and other aggressive treatments on frail elders. She introduces the subject gradually and carefully explains how aggressive, life-prolonging treatments can also compromise quality of life and prolong suffering. In addition, Marina asks if Dr. Rosenzweig and her son have ever thought about these issues or discussed them in the past with other health care providers.

As the discussion progresses, Dr. Rosenzweig's demeanor changes drastically: She gets visibly upset and explains to Marina that she has spent her whole life treating patients and has never asked "such stupid or thoughtless questions." She exclaims that she, like all good physicians, always did everything she could to save her patients. She also tells Marina how she was devoted to her own mother and did everything she could for her until her mother died at a very old age. Marina tries to appeal to Dr. Rosenzweig's son, expecting at least some understanding from him since he is a practicing physician in the United States. However, he only looks very uncomfortable and declines to take part in the conversation. Clearly, he is reluctant to participate in any decision making and does not want to discuss end-of-life issues. Marina has no choice but to document that the family elects to have full-code treatment.

Question:

1. What strategy would you develop to keep provider-patient communication open and create an environment conducive to educating older Russian-speaking Americans and their families on end-of-life issues?

Over the next few days after her admission, Dr. Rosenzweig sulks and declines to talk to Marina. Her son is also not approachable. As time goes by, Dr. Rosenzweig becomes accustomed to living in the facility and gradually warms up to Marina. They interact on many occasions but never again discuss end-of-life decisions.

For the next 4 years, Dr. Rosenzweig's residence at the facility is relatively uneventful. She gets sick often but bounces back with aggressive treatment. Eventually, she develops a viral pneumonia. As she and her son have requested, Dr. Rosenzweig receives all possible treatment but does not respond well. The team on the floor try to feed her and urge her to drink more fluids, but she refuses. Instead, she asks to talk to Marina and explains that she is suffering and wants to die peacefully without any more intervention. Dr. Rosenzweig dies within 2 days.

References

Aroian KJ, Khatutsky G, Tran TV, et al. Health and social service utilization among elderly immigrants from the former Soviet Union. *J Nurs Scholarsh* 2001;33(3):265–271.

Aroian KJ, Norris AE. Somatization and depression among former Soviet immigrants. *J Cult Diversity* 1999;6(3):93–101.

Aroian KJ, Spitzer A, Bell M. Family support and conflict among former Soviet immigrants. *West J Nurs Res* 1996;18(6):655–674.

Brod M, Heurtin-Roberts S. Older Russian emigres and medical care. *West J Med* 1992;157:333–336.

Farone S. Psychiatry and political oppression in the Soviet Union. *Amer Psychologist* 1982;37(10):1105–1112.

Smith L. New Russian immigrants: health problems, practices, and values. *J Cult Diversity* 1996;3(3):68–73.

Strumpf NE, Glicksman A, Goldberg-Glen R, et al. Caregiver and elder experiences of Cambodian, Vietnamese, Soviet Jewish, and Ukrainian refugees. *Int J Aging Hum Dev* 2001;53(3):243–262.

Tran TV, Khatutsky G, Aroian KJ, et al. Living arrangements, depression, and health status among elderly Russian immigrants. *J Gerontol Soc Work,* 2000;33(2):63–77.

Vishnevsky A, Zayonchkovskaya Z. Emigration from the former Soviet Union: the fourth wave. In: Fassman H, Munz R, eds. *European Migration in the Late Twentieth Century: Historical Patterns, Actual Trends, and Social Implications.* Brookfield, VT: Edward Elger Publishing Co.; 1994:239–285.

Wei C, Spigner C. Health status and clinic utilization among refugees from Southeast Asia and the Former Soviet Union. *J Health Education* 1994;25 (3):266–273.

Wheat ME, Brownstein H, Kvitash V. (1983). Aspects of medical care of Soviet Jewish émigrés. *West J Med* 1983;139(6):900–904.

INDEX

This index covers Volume I and II of Doorway Thoughts. The page numbers are preceded by "I" or "II" to indicate in which volume the topic appears.

CREDITS

Chapter Opener 2 © and images/Digital Vision Limited/age
                fotostock
Chapter Opener 3 © Adams Picture Library t/a apl/Alamy Images
Chapter Opener 4 © BlueMoon Stock/Alamy Images
Chapter Opener 5 © Digital Vision Limited/Getty Images
Chapter Opener 6 © Photodisc
Chapter Opener 7 © PhotoAlto/Jupiterimages
Chapter Opener 8 © ImageSource/age fotostock
Chapter Opener 9 © Mateusz Zagorski/ShutterStock, Inc.

The above images comprise the collages found on the cover and
Chapter Opener 1.

American Geriatrics Society
The American Geriatrics Society (AGS) is a nationwide, not-for-profit association of geriatric health care professionals dedicated to improving the health, independence, and quality of life for all older people. The AGS promotes high quality, comprehensive, and accessible health care for America's older population, including those who are chronically ill and disabled. The Society provides leadership to health care professionals, policy makers, and the public by developing, implementing, and advocating programs in patient care, research, professional and public education, and public policy.